The Mind Whisperer

Deeper Than a Whisper

Erotic Hypnosis 2.0
Sensual Trance and Beyond
Advanced Hypnotic Techniques for Multiple Contexts
(Therapy, Entertainment, and Adult Recreation)
2020 version update
Of
THE MIND WHISPERER

Cricket Press first published 2013/revised and updated 2020

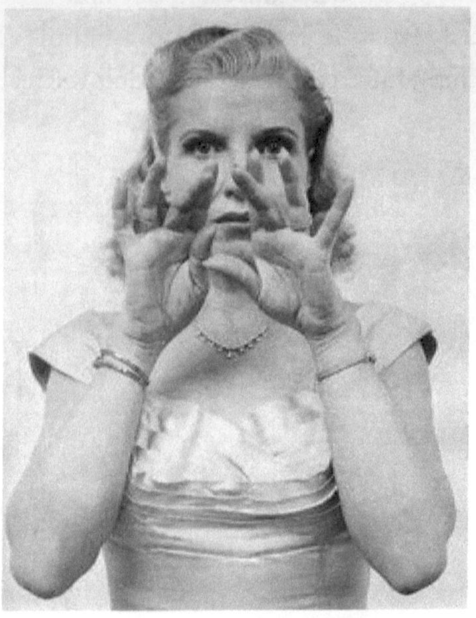

Dedication

The following people have been integral to the writing and development of this project, I would like to thank them all:

My parents, for not sending me away to a boy's home as they often threatened;

The pig, *who taught me to fly like an eagle.*

All the girls I've known before.

Every student who attended one of my workshops then thought the manual would make a really good book.

DEEPER THAN A WHISPER
Erotic Hypnosis 2.0
Sensual Trance and Beyond
Advanced Hypnotic Techniques for Multiple Contexts
(Therapy, Entertainment, and Adult Recreation)

Note: this manual was originally designed to accompany a program of lessons, taught in a workshop environment. While you will get a full education from the book, it is always better to have the experience of the class where each of these techniques can be demonstrated and experienced.

2020/2024 notes,

After much thought I have decided to upgrade this work, in the ensuring years since 2013 I have learned a lot more about life the universe and everything. While this book still contains all the original ideas and concepts it also contains a lot more. It is written in a more adult frame of mind. Basically, this means that as well as the new stuff, there is also a lot that I did not put in the original work as I felt at the time it was too sensitive, too confronting or perhaps political correctness stayed my hand. I've decided to go all out in this volume leaving no stone unturned. As I imagine anyone reading this book will want the full meat of the program. Finally, I discovered my book on torrent and other rip-off websites. So, in order to give value to those who are happy to invest in this book I rewrote the bulk of it.

Erotic hypnosis is a collection of hypnotic techniques for influencing or persuading a willing subject, (usually the submissive or slave ;) an agreed upon mind control using hypnosis to affect another person's sexuality or to alter the sexual perceptions of the subject, to enhance their sexual experiences or to aid in overcoming sexual dysfunctions.

Paraphrased from Wikipedia

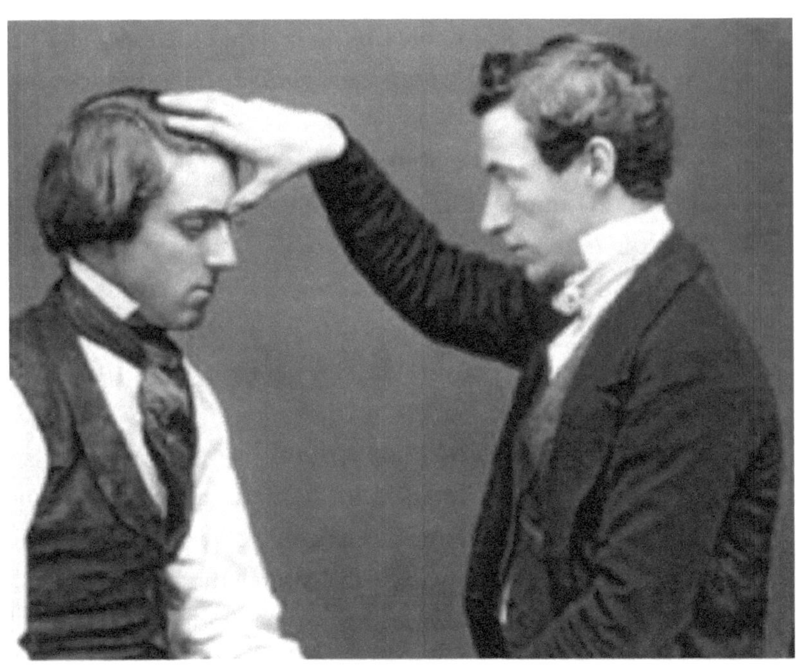

In 2013 when I first wrote this book, I said the following

Some professional hypnotists are going to hate this book for two reasons:

"First, it doesn't say enough. I have left out many important things due to timing and publication issues, plus this book was written for entertainment. The second reason they are going to dislike it is because I give away too much. The astute reader will see things or discover techniques that are long held, closely guarded secrets that many hypnotists do not want the run of the mill Joe Public to know.

So be astute dear reader...be astute.

In this 2020/2024 update a lot has been added, for example I left out some very powerful influencing principles with advanced rapport building techniques which I simply did not want to share. Along with the more erotic scripts. My original reasons have changed, so I will be sharing them in the book. Also, money was a constraint, I believe in value for money thus I tried to keep the cost for the reader reasonable that is no longer an issue, as I now believe that if you want this book, you will be happy to pay for it.

HYPNOSIS IS ACTUALLY ABOUT CONFIDENCE

Be confident. Possibly the most highly guarded secret of hypnotists is that Hypnosis is about belief. If someone believes that you can hypnotise them, they're already halfway there.

Your subject should have full confidence in you as a hypnotist, they should **believe** that you can hypnotize them.

When first starting out with your subject, do not act as if you are experimenting on them, or using them to gauge your learning or effectiveness.

Be confident. **Assume** that if you use the techniques correctly then the subject will become hypnotized no matter what. Treat it as a matter of course, then they will treat it that way as well.

A good technique to employ on your subject is to prepare a week or so ahead. Tell them you are going to learn hypnosis for their benefit, then after you have learned all you need to know, you will be back to place them in a trance. Wait about a week, or even two, then say, "Ok, I've learned the first part; I'm now going to hypnotize you."

Do not say, "Let's *try* this and see how it goes," or "can I *please try* to put you in a trance?" You must give the illusion that you can do it, that you're an expert at it, that it will work.

Another tack is to say nothing about learning or being a beginner. Just tell them you are a hypnotist. Sort of giving the impression that you have been for a long time, that you know exactly what you're doing, saying it with confidence, with surety. Your subject will assume that you are. The effect is similar to when some tells you they are a doctor, a veterinarian or a nurse... you instantly assume they are...

Remember hypnosis is about belief. Something I learned very early on in performing my stage shows is that if the audience doesn't believe you, then even the best techniques in the world won't help you. An audience sees my posters up at least three weeks before a show or reads the advertising; they assume that I must be able to hypnotize them, because otherwise I wouldn't have the posters with my picture on them.

This creates the belief (we call this *Pre-framing*) that I can do what I claim, therefore half the work is already done. A person who believes that you can hypnotize them is already half hypnotized.

This idea of *assumption* is a very powerful technique that we will discuss in detail later.

WHAT IF THEY DON'T WAKE UP?

Don't worry they will, the first thing to realise is that technically being hypnotised is not being asleep so there is nothing to wake up from. The subject is merely concentrating to the point where they become temporarily unaware of what's going on around them. Entering an altered state where unimportant things drift away, while important things like your voice and suggestions are focused on intently.

If perchance someone does refuse to wake up … just leave them, they will eventually fall into normal sleep, waking up normally, never panic or slap them out of it, you'll likely give them a heart attack.

Another good technique is to simply tell them that if they don't wake up something bad will happen, like we are all going off to the best party ever, if you stay here asleep you'll miss out. In my clinic I have just once said to a tranced client that *it's ok for you to stay here relaxing and deep asleep, in fact stay as long as you want it's only ten dollars per minute to keep enjoying this time.* The client opened his eyes immediately after that.

So remember you can't get "stuck" in hypnosis in the same way your subject can't get jammed awake or trapped in wakefulness.

KEYS TO A SUCCESSFUL INDUCTION

As stated earlier, it's really not that hard to get someone into the state of trance once you understand what's really occurring in the mind of the subject.

Because most people are already in some state of trance. Either very mild or fully intense, you are actually taking something that is a perfectly natural process, such as when we focus on a good book or movie.

You are using that natural state to cause the deeper hypnotic state. The human mind is already prone to 'zone out' under certain conditions. All that the hypnotist is doing, at a basic level, is using this natural tendency of the mind, to create an enhanced state of hyper focus.

Once the mind is in this state, it is more accepting of certain suggestions, the hypnotist is feeding his own suggestions into the subconscious, using terms or phrases that the mind will accept as correct or true, or that the mind has no objection to reacting to.

For example: next time someone is watching a movie notice when they become really intent on the story or the action to the point where they lean forward in their chair. You will notice that they themselves are not aware of the leaning forward, they have forgotten about their own bodies, focusing attentively on the movie. As a hypnotist you would make them aware of their bodies again by pointing out that they are leaning forward. Instantly two things occur in the subjects mind.

One: they become aware of their own feelings and the position of their body, Two: they are listening to you... you momentarily have taken control over what they are thinking and feeling.

Think about this right now! Your feet. Were you aware of them are you aware of them now?

At a more advanced level you will learn to give suggestions that are confusing to the subject's conscious mind. Suggestions that only the subconscious understands. In fact the subconscious may even feel *obligated* to follow certain suggestions if they are delivered in the right way.

So that's basically it...BELIEF IS THE KEY ... it's as simple as getting your subject believing in you while having confidence in yourself. While all this sounds simple enough, there is an art, a science to it that can take many years of practice to get really good at it. The subject must believe that you can hypnotize them; this is no different than going to a movie believing that you are going to enjoy it or going to a restaurant that has been recommended by friends. If you believe something, then your belief flavours how you react to it. If you have twenty friends, tell you that a certain restaurant sucks, then you won't go to eat there. If you believe that Joe can't hypnotize you, then why would you even bother to allow Joe to try?

However, there is still a lot you can do at the beginning stages of your training, then as you progress with practice, experience and a lot of study, anyone can become a good hypnotist.

SUGGESTIBILITY TESTS AND CONVINCERS,

Convincers are also known as Suggestibility Tests. They serve the triple purpose of

Testing That The Subject Is Willing To Go Into Hypnosis

At The Same Time Convincing Them That They Can Be Hypnotised

While Installing The Belief That You Are A Capable Hypnotist.

Creating the belief in your subject is the first key to successfully hypnotizing them. You must create a situation where they have, at the very least, confidence that you are able to cause "something" to happen. This is why we use **convincers;** (suggestibility tests) they are designed to convince the subject that you are a hypnotist, and that they can be hypnotized.

Later we will examine a series of well-known, effective convincers, but for the moment let's look at *how* they work.

What's really happening during the **test** is an examination of your subject's willingness to allow you to hypnotise them.

Suppose that you are in situation where you are called upon to show your amazing skills as a hypnotist. You offer to demonstrate, a volunteer steps forward. You stand them up straight, say a few words, telling them (*Strongly Suggesting*) that they won't be able to open their eyes. Suddenly they can't. They try harder but still they can't open their eyes. Is it magic or did you hypnotize them? Either way, they are now convinced that you know what you're talking about, you can indeed do what you claimed.

During this process you have actually done several things. You have secured some very important information.

Firstly this person was willing to volunteer, therefore they are likely to also be willing to go into full trance state. They are suggestible

Second, they will follow orders.

Thirdly. You have made them believe that something happened, that you are responsible for making it happen.

Having created the belief that you are indeed capable of hypnotizing people, the next step is inducing a trance. The subject now has increased confidence that if they sit in the chair listening to you, stare into your eyes or watch the watch, they will become hypnotized.

So now you actually hypnotize them; as stated before, you are simply using the natural tendency of the human mind *to zone out* to create the first stage of hypnosis or the hypnotic trance state. This is called the *induction*.

There are several good inductions in this book, including a few of my own design, which have been developed over many years of working with clients or stage performances.

Years of experience have shown me powerful methods of moving from the testing or convincer stage into the induction stage in a smooth even flow.

There are rapid inductions, instant inductions plus a variety of normal inductions, all of which use the normal natural stages that a mind will go through, either in the shock state, the normal sleeping state or focusing state.

An important note. The sciences of psychology and hypnosis have come a long way in the last few decades. Almost no hypnotist today will take out an old fob watch waving it about to induce trance; he may cause a *Fixation Effect* with a pen or his ring, but rarely a watch.

As you practice the various inductions one very important thing will happen: *you are going to discover your own ways of inducing trance*. It may be word based, (linguistics) where you use hypnotic statements or phrasing; it may be voice based, using the cadence of your voice, or it may involve fixation methods. It may even be a blend of these, based on your personality, natural gifts with your practised talents, which you will develop as you learn the process.

I think I can safely assume that you have some natural talent or desire in the area of hypnosis or mind control. Otherwise you wouldn't be reading this book.

Not too many years ago, hypnosis was about the supposed influence of the hypnotist; today it is about the willingness of the subject. Those old 1950's suspense movies have a lot to answer for; they created the illusion that hypnotists had some mysterious occult power. Today we know that it is actually the subject allowing themselves to be hypnotized. (*Applied willingness*) Understanding this simple fact alone can make you a better, more effective hypnotist.

The next key to a great induction is your linguistics how you apply *words*, or *language patterns.* This is possibly the hardest part of the process for the novice hypnotist, I suggest you study NLP or listen very carefully to virtually every word you say during the induction. In fact, I highly recommend that you record your first few practice inductions then play them back, listening very carefully for the effect your words might have on your subject.

Better than this is to pay attention to how you use language or communicate in all situations.

Often when we speak, we are full of contradictions, misplaced words or sentences that don't make sense, in normal conversation, people are very forgiving.

In our rush to be heard we let most of these slip past our awareness. In the hypnotic state however, the mind of the subject becomes incredibly focused on every word you say.

If you say something confusing or untrue, the subject may question this in their mind, then not listen to your next statement, or snap out of trance altogether, thus you will lose them.

Let's suppose you're telling your subject, in the erotic situation, that they are a famous porn star, there is a very good chance that your subject will feel they are ***not*** a famous porn star. They may be shy, have self-image issues because they are overweight or afraid to act out such fantasies. It just may not fit them well, they may subconsciously start going against the suggestion.

Keep this in mind as we progress!

THE NEXT KEY IS THE DEEPENER.

Having successfully tested then taken the subject into trance, you will want to proceed into a deeper state of hypnosis, the state where you are able to make suggestions that the subconscious will act on. To go to this level we use ***deepeners***.

There are several in the book that will enable you to take your subject to the somnambulistic state. Deepeners are going to be especially important for your erotic hypnosis to work.

Taking the subject to this state, to a place they enjoy, where they fully experience the effects, will require you to have a clear understanding of how deepeners work on the psyche.

All this means nothing, however, unless you understand what your subject expects from the hypnotic sessions, especially with older, more educated people. Many people will already have some idea of what they think hypnosis is; if you do something in the induction stage or the deepening stage that conflicts with this idea, again you are likely to lose them.

The greatly respected Gerald K describes it this way, *"**There are The Four Mental Attitudes that the hypnotist must take into account when designing his or her suggestions. When an individual is in hypnosis and hears a suggestion they will take one of four mental attitudes about that suggestion. The mental attitude the*** *subject takes will determine whether the suggestion is accepted or rejected. The subject has no alternative but to choose one of the following states of mind:"*

1. *"I like that suggestion. I know it's going to work for me!"*
2. *"I don't know; it sounds a little uncomfortable to me. It just doesn't fit me."*
3. *"I'm neutral about it. I don't care if I get it or don't get it."*
4. *"I like that suggestion. I hope it works!"*

"The only mental attitude that will cause the suggestion to be accepted is #1. Any other will cause the suggestion to be rejected and there will be no change. In short the process must make sense to the subject".

This is why Pre-Talk or safety talk is so important. It's called a safety talk **not** because it details all the dangers of hypnosis but because it makes it safe for you to hypnotize the subject. It is designed as a safety or explanation talk.

Stage hypnotists have been using it for years, we each develop our own style of delivering it. The point, as far as the audience is concerned, is that you are showing and explaining that hypnosis is safe, that it can be a lot of fun. While this is true, there is another level of work going on, the hypnotist is mentally preparing his audience to accept that whatever he says is hypnosis actually is hypnosis.

For example, in my opening stage talk I use a phrase very similar to one above, *"hypnosis has come a long way in the last few year; I won't be using a watch to hypnotize anyone here tonight."*

If anyone in the audience had actually been expecting me to wave a watch about, now they aren't. Also, I haven't told them what I will do, or how I'm going to induce the state of hypnosis. Therefore anything I say or do could, as far as they are concerned, be hypnosis.

As long as it looks and feels like I'm doing something that could hypnotize them, is congruent and makes sense. Even though they may not fully understand the process, they will assume that I do understand it, because I am, after all, the hypnotist.

I use similar ideas in my clinical work, I might say something to the effect of well today I'm going to hypnotise you, I will give you a few relaxation excersisies.to see how you go... after this point the client will assume that what's happening is about relaxation

Thus it will be with you, when you have that first subject in the chair; if they believe you can do it, any expectations they may have of what it might look like or feel like to be hypnotized are vague, you already have them in a state of belief, so they are effectively already in a state of hypnosis. Mild as it might be, they are already hypnotized.

WHAT HAVE WE LEARNED SO FAR?

Belief: creating beliefs about hypnosis, or working with the subject's existing beliefs about hypnosis. Or creating an atmosphere that is conducive to hypnosis.

Convincing: convincing the subject that

a) You are a capable hypnotist,

b) That they can be hypnotised.

Induction: putting the subject into the hypnotic state.

Deepener: making that hypnotic state into a full workable trance, where the subject will suspend rationale doing what you ask them.

Now let's break that up into usable parts.

In the highly technical world of hypnotherapy, convincers are sometimes referred to as ***suggestibility tests.*** They are used to test the suggestibility level of subjects. However, for the purpose of this book, we will treat them as both tests of suggestibility as well as techniques for convincing a subject that you can hypnotize them.

Convincers work on multiple levels. First, they convince the subject that you are able to hypnotize them, confirming that they can be placed under the influence of your words or techniques.

More importantly, a well delivered convincer enables you to directly place commands in the subject's mind that they must follow. This is sometimes referred to as pre-framing or pre-hypnotising. In effect you are actually hypnotising the subject ahead of when they think you are going to hypnotise them.

A good convincer puts you in command of the situation, the process creates a position of authority getting the subject following your orders from the outset. Generally without them being aware that you are doing this. It becomes perfectly natural for them to do as you command.

Understanding this is going to be a great assistance later when we discuss **Covert** or **Hidden Hypnosis Tactics,** because a good convincer can actually hypnotize someone.

Convincers also have a certain wow factor that I enjoy. Anyone watching you do convincers on someone will assume that you are exhibiting some sort of '***Power of Influence***" they will think you are actually hypnotizing the subject. Many times the subject themselves will laugh awkwardly or feel amazed that you were able to manipulate or influence them in such a way. My personal convincers involve a fair bit of advanced NLP with surreptitious hypnosis strategy, they have taken me years to perfect. I'll alleviate the pain of you learning them by trial and error, giving you the standard convincers used by hypnotists, then my reworking of them, then we will examine them in the erotic context.

Finally, *never ever* refer to convincers *as* convincers; act as if they are part of the hypnotic process. In fact, if you treat these convincers as if they were a natural part of how you hypnotize a subject, that is what they will become, rather than just convincing, you will actually be hypnotizing your subject as you convince them.

With practise you will be able to tell when the subject has reached compliance, as soon as you get that compliance, move straight into an induction.

Do these well then soon you'll find yourself being invited to a lot more parties! You might also want to check out this video on my channel

HYPNO HISTORY 1

https://www.youtube.com/watch?v=xtawB7aDED0&t=1s

CONVINCERS AND TESTING
EYES WIDE SHUT OR EYES LOCKED

As far as I know, there are two old, very popular convincers; these are *the hands locked together* and *the eyes locked shut* suggestibility tests.

Basically, you are convincing the subject that they cannot open their eyes, until you give them permission to do so. Many hypnotherapist use this technique as a test of the subject's suggestibility, because that is exactly what it is.

On stage, if the chosen subject does not do as instructed, I proceed no further with them, moving on instead to the next subject. As a rule, I will use three convincers before I am persuaded that a subject will *not* go into trance. That said, however, I have often found that the first subject will see the other volunteers on stage behaving correctly then start to fall into the trance state themselves. (Peer pressure can be very powerful)

Unlike stage work though, when hypnotizing the individual, whatever happens is going to be correct. This also works in therapy, even if they do open their eyes, you will be able to use this as part of the process. I will explain this in greater depth later.

Finally, even though I am presenting the convincers in a particular order, you don't have to do them in any specific order, in fact you don't even need to do all of them. Depending on your experience with the willingness of your subject, you only ever need to do one or two convincers. The theory being that the more you know and understand them, the more you learn to observe the subtlest reactions of a subject the more fun they can be, the more effective you will be as a hypnotist.

THE OLD METHOD

(Place your right thumb slightly above the bridge of the subject's nose applying slight pressure) about where the third eye is supposed to be.

Say the following...

"I'm going to count from five down to one. As I do, your eyelids will lock so tightly closed that the more you try to open them, the tighter they're locking closed.

Five, your eyes are pressing down tightly.

Four, pressing down and sealing shut.

Three, sealing as if they are glued.

Two, they're locked shut. The more you try to open them, the tighter they're locking closed.

One, Okay, try to open your eyelids now, and find them locking tighter and tighter. That's fine. You can stop trying now. Just relax and go deeper."

THE NEW METHOD

I cannot stress enough that as a hypnotist, every word you say is of the utmost importance. You must carefully structure what you are saying to make sense within the mind of the subject.

Your wording must be measured to bypass the **Critical Reasoning Factor** of your subject. Simply stating, "When I count to five, your eyes will be locked shut," will only work after a person is fully hypnotized, or not at all. You must convince them, hence the name of this process.

Here is an advanced way of doing the eyes shut test that takes into account all we have learned thus far:

Have the subject sit down. Make sure that the atmosphere of the room is right for hypnosis. If you're at a party where get called upon to demonstrate, either decline politely or change something. Get the host to lower the lights or put on some meditation music, anything that changes the atmosphere of the room, making it more seductive or hypnotic.

Once the subject is seated, you will sit facing them. Tell you're volunteer to sit up with their back straight, hands on their lap. This is a **Direct Command**, in reality there is no real reason they need to be in this position. You are saying this to get them to obey your commands, to make it normal for them to do as you instruct, so deliver these instructions in a firm, yet friendly, almost casual tone.

If standing, use a firm yet pleasant voice, say something to the effect of "Now stand here, feet together, hands by your side and look, stare, straight ahead".

Don't say, "**Please** stand here. Now, would you **please** place your hands at your side, or whatever is comfortable?"

This is not a direct command. You must get the subject used to the idea, through your language, that you are directing them.

You never make this obvious; it's just the way it is, you are the expert they must follow your directions to be hypnotized, to enjoy the experience.

Although it is never actually stated this way, you make it so though actions and your positive commanding presence. In reality, it doesn't matter if the subject sits stands or lies down; it's about them following your orders or instructions.

Once you have them in a comfortable place, reach across start gently tapping the subject's forehead just above and between the eyes, where the third eye is traditionally found. This should be an unperceivable gentle tapping almost a caress. As you do this, simply say:

"Now just do exactly as I say, follow my instructions and I promise you'll feel awesome and you'll go into deep trance"

"Now close those eyes. Just let them close."

This should be a gentle, yet no-nonsense tone, as if you've done it a thousand times before, as if you fully expect those eyes to close as you command it.

The astute reader will notice that we did not say, "Now let *"your"* eyes close." There is a very important reason for this, as every single word in this testing convincer has been very carefully put in place for maximum effect.

Using the statement **"those eyes"** creates **Disassociation** in the mind of the subject, where one might resist closing his or her own eyes, there is less resistance in allowing another far away set of eyes to close. It's almost like imagining somebody else letting their eyes shut down, tight, heavy and relaxed.

The second part is also important; *just let them close* takes away responsibility and control from the subject. In one sense you are saying, "don't control it, and don't *make* them close, just *let* them close in response to me and what I'm doing."

Again, this instantly (in most cases) dissociates the subject, they assume on a subconscious level that you, the hypnotist are somehow making their eyes close. They are convincing themselves that you are hypnotizing them.

Now continue gently tapping the forehead of the subject and say:

"As I do this, you notice how easy it is to concentrate and focus. You notice that you can concentrate more easily, think a bit more clearly, focus. As you focus on my voice just roll your eyes up, as if you could see my fingertip through your skull; in fact, imagine that you can."

"And as you continue to focus and concentrate on my voice and these directions, you will notice a very strange thing. In a moment, when I count down from five to one, you will be unable to open your eyes. It will be as if they are stuck shut, as if your eyelids are glued down, tightly shut. In fact, the harder you try to open them, the more tightly they will stick together, shutting tightly. Try as you might, you can't open them. The more you try, the more tightly closed locked they become. It may be that they have relaxed so much that you just don't want to open them, that you just can't be bothered. They feel so heavy and relaxed and comfortable that you just don't want to open them; that they are just kind of drifting off to sleep. You may notice that they are so relaxed, heavy and

comfortable that they just don't want to open, so by the time I count down to five just let them go. They become so heavy, so relaxed, so tightly stuck down, that you can't open them; that you won't open them.

Five

Eyes still turned upward, looking up, focusing, and concentrating on my voice and my suggestions.

Four

Those eyes completely closed. So tight, so relaxed, heavy and restful, that you can't open them. They just don't want to open. The harder you try to, the more tightly shut they become. The muscles working against you, locking them down as you let go.

Three

Down, deeper and deeper; relaxing more and letting go with each breath, with each number down. It's almost as if the muscles of the eyes and around the eyes act independently of you, shutting down, locking tighter and tighter, heavier and more relaxed.

Two

You will try, but you won't open them. Try harder, but they shut down even tighter. The harder you try, the more they will refuse to open.

One

Locked so tightly now, that even as you attempt to open them, they shut tighter. Try, but you can't open them.

Wait a moment then:

Ok, 1, 2, 3. You can open them, open your eyes now.

It is not hard to see how this breaks down into the hypnotic effect, how the hypnotist is directing the thought processes of the subject. For example, there is a disconnection created that separates the eyelids from the person, almost implying that they, by themselves, don't want to open them.

Let's examine a few of the effects that occur in this test...

"Or it may be that they have relaxed so much that you just don't want to open them, that you can't be bothered."

Here you are also giving the subject more than one option, either their eyes will be stuck down by force, or they will be so relaxed that they simply won't want to open. This also causes slight confusion within the subject. This is a **Controlled Confusion** it is done for a purpose. When the mind is confused it will tend to go back to the last thing it understood, the last thing it was *not* confused about. Or hook onto the next thing it hears.

You will notice that immediately before or after each of these confusing statements there was something that the mind of the subject could understand, the direct order that the eyes won't open. *"You will try but you won't open them."*

We also discovered the "**as if**" effect here, this is a way of allowing the subject to give themselves permission to follow the commands, as with the line, "*as if* the eyelids are glued down."

It was simply snuck in, in such a way that it bypassed the critical part of the mind, the part of the mind that says, "Wait a minute, there's no real glue here, my eyes aren't stuck down at all."

I came across this effect in the early days of my stage work. I would have a volunteer become Elvis Presley. The audiences loved seeing their mates acting out the role, however, every once in a while, somebody would not do it; they wouldn't follow the suggestion.

I finally figured out that it was the way I was **giving the suggestion.** Instead of saying "*you will be Elvis,*" I changed the line to "*it will be as if you have become Elvis.*"

It's safer for the subject, as it allows the **pretend part of the mind** to activate to be "as if." There is little to no argument with the statement. Instead of the rational part of the mind saying, "Ok I'm not Elvis, Elvis is dead. I can't suddenly turn into Elvis. This is bullshit."

It instead reasons, "***Ok I can pretend to be Elvis. That's Ok; I'm just acting out a role.***"

You will also notice that toward the end of the test the hypnotist says "***so by the time I count down to five, just let them go. They become so heavy, so relaxed, so tightly stuck down, that you can't open them; that you won't open them.***"

This is a subtle way of slipping in the command that they won't open them. It's actually a hidden instruction not to open their eyes; you are telling the subject that they ***won't*** do it.

It subconsciously connects to the opening lines about following your directions exactly.

Finally, this is a ***Psychophysical Effect***, partly caused by the fact that it is very difficult to open your eyes while looking up through the skull. You of course do not tell the subject this, you allow them to assume its hypnosis that assumption leads to belief, and belief leads to actual hypnosis...

There is no need to remember this eyes wide shut routine verbatim. In fact, of the thousand or more times I've done it, I'm certain it has never been the same twice. What is important is that you understand the principals involved.

These are...

The True Purpose of the Testing Phase

Getting the Subject to Comply With Your Commands
The Disconnecting or Disassociation of the Person from the Eyes
Methods of Hiding Your Commands
Providing More Than One Reason for an Effect to Work
The As If Effect Allowing the Subject to Be Ok With Your Suggestions

These suggestibility tests, or convincers, can be an art form in themselves. Practise them. After a while you may even surprise yourself at how changing a few simple words, how structuring your speech into patterns can have a profound effect on anyone listening.

Later, in the advanced section, you are going to learn a much more powerful **language set** that creates instant hypnosis, with the eyes wide shut convincer. It will go in the first part as follows:

"As I do this, you will probably notice how easy you can concentrate and focus. You might notice that parts of you are already beginning to relax, that you can concentrate more easily, think just a bit more clearly, relax just a little more deeply. Focus on my voice, and as you focus on my voice you find yourself relaxing even more deeply. Just let your eyes roll up; as if you could see my finger through your skull, in fact imagine that you can."

The changes are subtle, yet the effect is powerful it will help you lead the subject from the testing stage through to the induction stage in one clean movement.

We will now look at another convincer or suggestibility test, adding more principles to the ones we have just learned.

SPINNING HANDS

In this convincer, we will be applying some of the things we have already learned, also I will be introducing a few new concepts.

Have the subject sit, with you standing behind them, leaning forward to speak directly (yet softly) into their ear.

"This time I'm going behind you to raise your hands."

Reach around bringing the subject's hands up to about chest level. This is the **anchoring stage,** which I will explain later.

"Now start moving them around each other."

This is a rolling motion. Start spinning their hands around each other showing them how you want them to move their hands.

"Now, as I release your hands, continue the motion of your own accord."

Release their hands.

"Just let them go. It's as if they are doing it all by themselves. Moving, spinning, turning. Moving, spinning, turning. Even faster now. Moving, spinning, turning. That's good.

As your hands are turning, I want you to think about your heart. Your heart beats automatically in response to the needs of your body. In the same way, your hands are turning automatically, so that the more you try to stop the motion, the faster they turn.

I'm going to touch your forehead. The instant I do, your hands spin in the opposite direction."

Touch or just gently tap the subject's forehead.

"Back the other way, moving, spinning, and turning. And as they're turning, you're going much deeper in relaxation. This time, as I touch your forehead, your left arm drops limply down to your side; your right arm continues the movement."

Touch their forehead.

"Left arm drops; right arm continues, and as it's moving you're going deeper and deeper into hypnosis. This time when I touch your forehead, your right arm drops limply down. You go much deeper."

Touch their forehead.

"Drop it down and go deeper. That's fine."

This is a **Kinetic Testing Procedure** or convincer. It causes a contact with the body, the emotions the feelings of the subject. You may have already guessed, however, that there is a lot more going on here than is first seen.

When we think about it, there is no real reason to mention anything at all about the subject's heart rate. Yet by doing so you are causing a mental shift to the internal state: the subject thinks about his or her body, feels it, they become aware of it. Then while they are in that awareness you are able to draw them toward thinking that the body is relaxing. They will "***feel***" whatever you tell them to feel. Remember our example of the friend watching a movie and leaning forward!

The ***as if*** effect is delivered very subtly at this line, ***"Just let them go. It's as if they are doing it all by themselves."***

You are in effect saying, "I want you to pretend that your hands are spinning of their own volition."

You are also creating other important anchors; the touch to the forehead, the hands being held when you show the subject how they should spin are beautiful unexpected anchors. You are effectively telling the subject that touching them means they will obey you. In erotic hypnosis this is very important. Later, when you want to cause a specific effect via a touch to the forehead, the shoulder or other part of the body, your subject will be pre-programmed (*sometimes called* **pre-framing**) to perceive that touch as the anchor to obey you. In other words, they know that when you touch them *something* is going to happen, you will have told them *what* is going to happen.

So you are setting up all the mental procedures you need for induction and post hypnotic suggestion stages in the experience.

Here is a spooky hypnotic effect you can perform at parties when it becomes obvious that you are a hypnotist, when somebody says "hey do some of your Hypno Stuff for us" have everyone sit facing you, look at each person in the eyes, quickly scanning the room ... put a hypnotic look on your face... now say

"I want you all to concentrate on the back of your neck, can you feel the warmth, feel it getting warmer, raise your hand if you can feel the warmth growing at the back of your neck now"...

Almost everyone will raise their hand.

Why because you have drawn attention to the back of the neck, it's always warm, it helps regulates body temperature, this is a Psychophysical *Effect* the back of our neck is always slightly warmer yet we are unaware of it, as with the spinning hands test you are making your subject pay attention to an area of the body we generally don't think about. By paying more attention to it they will notice the warmth. You of course will take credit for the effect!

The effect is similar to that create when we yawn, then other people yawn as well or when you create an itch in your subject simply by describing what an itch feels like.

HEAVY LIGHT HANDS

The following is one of my personal favourites. I use it during my stage show because it is fun, it allows me to take an entire audience on the journey. I don't have to judge reactions or choose who is compliant; the audience does this themselves, then they willingly walk on stage becoming part of the show.

That said, it is also a well-known effective one-on-one test as well. In fact, it was originally a suggestibility test for a single subject, which I adapted for my stage show. It also a good place to teach our next couple of hypnotic principles, the **out breath** and using *language to create effective images*.

Have the subject sit facing you.

Have them close their eyes.

Pre-talk (or set the subject up) as follows:

"Don't worry, I'm not hypnotising you just yet. This is a test of the imagination, your ability to visualise and believe. And the more you visualise, the more effective this will be. The more you believe and follow my suggestions, the more fun we will have with this and the more real it will feel.

Now reach out take both the subject's hands (anchoring) raise them to just below shoulder level, saying the following:

"Now as you relax, (Let go of the subject's hands they should keep them outstretched, if not tell them to just keep them there) *and as you close those eyes... I want you to imagine and believe that on the back of your left hand I'm placing a book. It's a very heavy book, an encyclopaedia. And even as you begin to believe that, your arm becomes heavy, the weight of the book begins to feel very heavy. Your shoulder is aware of the weight of the book, and now your elbow and the back of the hand... feel that weight. It's heavy, uncomfortable and tiring."*

"Now on your right hand," (gently touch the back of the right hand, so they know what you're referring to, and to further anchor

the hands.) *"I am tying a balloon; the balloon is full of lighter than air gas, so it floats upward at the end of a string. Upwards... gently taking the left hand with it. Rising, lifting... upwards, while the right hand becomes heavier, more fatigued, tired, heavier and heavier ... being taken down by the weight of the book, as the left hand becomes lighter, raised up by the balloon. The right hands is heavy, the left hand is being elevated, taken upward by the gentle lifting of the balloon."*

Now continue in this fashion switching from the left hand to the right hand, reinforcing the heaviness or lightness of each hand, directing the hands up or down, heavier or lighter.

Now let's look at the hypnotic effects examining what is really occurring during this test.

THE OUT-BREATH TECHNIQUE

You will notice three dots ... at places during the convincer, later in scripts and inductions used in this book; these denote that you, the hypnotist, should wait until the subject is **breathing out** before delivering the next line.

This is a highly effective hypnotic technique that creates a state of relaxation for the subject. It does so using the natural physiological tendencies of the human body, when we breathe out, we are more relaxed than when we breathe in; it's a natural thing.

Try this experiment on your friends as well as your subjects, sit them down stare at them and say:

"Ok take a deep breath in for me. Now hold that breathe, and in a moment, I want you to just let the air out, in a sigh, just let it go... now let it go... And feel your shoulders relax and get heavy as you do this."

They will actually feel the shoulders relax and get heavy. This is a great way to begin any induction. More on this later; for now simply practise delivering your lines in a way that matches your important statements with the subject's outward breathing.

WORDING OR LANGUAGE

As I have stated, every word you say is important. Hypnosis is 80% language. During any test or induction, part of your task will be to choose words that are descriptive, exciting or different than your normal language. Words that create images or metaphors.

Do not fall into the trap of using plain and simple wording; during the test you will notice the words *raise, rise, lift, and elevate*. These are more descriptive ways of saying the same thing, allowing you the option of repeating a suggestion without appearing to be a parrot.

One of the golden rules of hypnosis when using **Post Hypnotic Suggestions** is to **repeat each suggestion at least three times**, more if you can. Rather than repeating the same thing over and over again, use different words or **Elegant Language**. You will find it more creative, a side effect of this is that the subject will focus more on what you're saying. More importantly, during the intermediate to advances stages of this work, you are going to learn a very important fact:

"THAT EVERY WORD YOU SAY HAS AN EFFECT ON THE PERSON HEARING IT".

This will become your mainstay as a hypnotist. I cannot emphasis this enough.

There is a part of the mind that is hard-wired to enjoy stories. As children, we enjoyed, even looked forward to hearing stories. The best stories are descriptive and exciting. Stories automatically place us in trance. So the more *story like* your tests, inductions or suggestions are, the more easily or readily they are accepted by the subconscious of your subject.

Another important thing to keep in mind is that *Implied Information* is more likely to enter the subconscious than direct information. More on this later.

THE FALLING TEST

Let's recap. We have learned that language is important, due to the psychology of the human mind. Some phrases are more hypnotic if delivered as the subject breathes out.

We have learned that directing the thoughts inward "feeling" is powerful. For example when you say just focus on your heart rate, your breathing, or the back of your neck, you are guiding the subject's thoughts to themselves. They will then pay attention to what they are experiencing. You can then tell them what to experience.

We have learned that storytelling is more effective than "***hey you, sleep***". (*Later I will show you how to make this effective as well.*)

The **Falling Test** is possibly the most famous of all the inductions or testing stages. You will have seen it in movies, on stage or in documentaries concerning our craft. Once again, however, there is a lot more going on than first meets the eye. We are going to use this convincer to more fully examine the ***Principle of Anchoring***.

Anchoring is a subtly powerful, effect way of controlling virtually anyone, even without hypnosis. It is, however, extremely powerful when combined with hypnotic suggestions or hypnotic language patterns.

A few things you need to know first,

A principle is more powerful than a technique, you can learn techniques until you are blue in the face then still not get it. Learn the principle behind it, then you will be able to create your own techniques. That is gold.

Anchoring is a way of ***Changing State***. A state is what a person feels or experiences in a given situation. When a man puts on his police uniform to go to work, his state changes from the weekend slob, drinking beer with his mates, to a figure of authority and determination. When a woman puts on perfume or lingerie, she changes state from a housewife to seductive temptress. When we change clothing we change state because clothing anchors that state.

Almost anything that comes into physical contact with our body can create an anchor of some type. Jewellery might make us feel more attractive, we actually *feel* it. A firm hand shake makes us feel confident either about ourselves or the person delivering it, it can determine who is in charge. When we are sad a cuddle makes us feel better, or it can release emotions, bringing us to tears.

In the ***Falling Test*** we are going to place anchors within the subject. This must be subtle. A technique I developed some years ago for this test along with a few other ways of installing anchors, is to tense the forearms not the fingers. By doing this the tension of the hands and fingers changes just outside the conscious perception of the subject.

Stand your subject in the middle of the room. Place yourself behind them directing them to look up at the wall, at the point where the wall meets the ceiling. Point at the place where you want them to look, as you direct them to the place you want them to stand, place your other hand briefly on your subjects shoulder.

"Ok, stand with your feet together, hands by your side and stare at the wall for me; just that point where the wall meets the ceiling, just focus your attention on that point...good."

Place a hand on each shoulder. As you point where you want them to look

"Ok, good, now focus."

Move the fingers to lightly rest on the temples of the subject, as if just adjusting the head to look upward in the right direction.

"Good, that's fine." Feet together hands by your side"

Let the fingers move away from the temples back to the shoulders.

"Now in a moment I'm going to place my fingers on your temples, at the side of your head, and we are going to use your imagination, possibly the most powerful thing you have,(now place your fingertips at the temples) *and you are going to imagine that in*

each of my fingertips is a powerful magnet,(start a gentle drawing back motion as if you almost want to pull them back) *a very powerful magnet, and in your temples are magnets, very powerful magnets, and you will feel a powerful attraction drawing you back. This magnetic attraction will be so powerful that it will draw you back. Don't worry, I won't let you fall. It will draw you backward so powerfully, and you will feel it, as if powerful magnets in my fingers and in your temples are drawing you backward, backward. The more you fight it, the stronger this magnetic force becomes... taking you back. A very powerful force, a magnet force, drawing you back."*

Your subject will teeter backward, ready to fall into your arms, don't let them fall; this would be impolite.

Now, the most powerful anchor, *as the subject falls back, you catch them at the shoulders say:*

"Don't worry you're safe."

Squeeze their shoulders, making it appear that you are helping them regain their footing.

You have just inserted a powerful, virtually permanent anchor that *in your presence, the subject is safe*. If you have done this correctly each time you touch or make contact with the subject's shoulders, they will feel safe even secure, they may even have the *sense* that you will stop them from falling.

You can extend the script as much as is suitable for your subject. The idea is to tell the subject they are falling backwards, due to the imaginary magnets combined with your hypnotic influence. Several things occur here; at certain key words you will ever so slightly tense the forearms creating an almost unperceivable change in the tension of the fingers against the forehead.

Those key words are setting up the anchor, which you will *fire* later. The key words are up to you; for me, they relate to any words that I might want to use later such as *"you will," "don't worry, I will catch you,"* or *"you will feel it."*

Essentially, any wording or language I intend to use later to get a reaction from the subject during hypnosis, where it is reasonable for me to touch the subject's shoulders or temples again, is an anchor.

Statements such as *"you will feel"* could, in the right context, be taken as direct commands, thus are appropriate for enhancing your anchors.

In the intermediate to advanced sections we will discuss anchors more fully; for the moment this should give you an understanding of how they work, in addition to how they can be applied.

HAND LEVITATION SUGGESTIBILITY TEST

The hand levitation is often used as a subtle way of moving your subject into hypnotic trance because it is easy for the subject to experience. In one sense the subject is in control, this can provide the hypnotist with many clues as to how the subject is progressing.

It also provides us with many opportunities to incorporate or practice a number of advanced techniques, including *Concentrated Attention* or *Absorption*, along with *Repetitive and Monotonous Stimulation*.

Hand Levitation is also a good stepping off point for *Post-Hypnotic Suggestions* which we will examine later.

The participant, while seated, looks at his or her resting hand concentrating on the idea that it will rise upward into the air a considerable distance without deliberately lifting it. The phenomenon consists of the *Subjectively Convincing Experience* of the hand rising upward against the direction of gravity without conscious voluntary action. (*In some cases this can be quite spooky*)

Subject is seated with hands resting on his or her lap

Just sit relax and let the eyes close. That's good. Now just bring your awareness to your right hand. Just think about it as you breath ... (remember to wait for the subject to be in the out breath)

38

just focus on it as each breath flows in...and out... letting each breath relax you ...deeply...and as you become more aware of your hand ,the wrist, the forearm, feeling it... becoming aware of it, how it feels as it just rests there, you might notice a heightened sense of awareness, perhaps you are aware of the muscles relaxing, from the fingers all the way up the forearm, perhaps this sensitivity makes you aware of the temperature of the air on your arm, and the small hairs on your arm, and as you focus on it how it feels, even where it is, you may notice a very strange thing, you may notice that your arm seems to be getting lighter, that's the weight is dissipating, shifting out of your arm, that the muscles are becoming lighter and lighter, that the arm is becoming so light that it begins to feel almost as if it is lifting ,,, raising upward like a balloon full of air, light and drifting upward ...

Continue until the subjects arm floats upward.

Don't worry if the subjects arm doesn't actually lift up; remember *Everything That Happens Is Correct For That Subject.* If the arm doesn't float after a reasonable time, bring them round asking *how did that feel?*

They will tell you that it felt as if the arm had become light they may even report that it felt like it was floating (even though it actually wasn't) nod your head knowingly saying, *good that's what was supposed to happen, your mind created the sensation, your subconscious made it feel as if your arm was floating, excellent work you will be a good subject.*

Continue on as if everything is normal.

Here is a good place to examine a few more details of the principles used. You will have noticed the phrase *"you may notice a very strange thing, you may notice that your arm seems to be getting lighter"* this is an *Erickson Technique* that almost forces the subject to notice exactly what you tell them to notice. Even if their arm isn't getting light, as soon as you say this they will actually pay attention to their arm with whatever feelings or sensations they notice, simply by paying more attention to it, will translate as a sense or feeling of lightness.

MAGNETIC FINGERS TEST

In the next convincer we will apply all we have learned plus discover a new very powerful application called the **Resistance Effect** or the **Try Effect**. Differing schools or books on hypnosis will have different names for it, yet the principle is the same. The harder one resists or *tries not to*, the harder it is not to.

Have the subject sit again facing you; have them interlock the fingers, extending the two pointer fingers apart.

Nine times out of ten the subject will look down paying attention to their fingers, this is what you want, if they don't tell them to *"look down and focus on your fingers"*

Now say the following or your version of it.

"Just imagine that your fingers contain powerful magnets... and even as you begin to believe this your fingers are drawn together by the magnets ... powerful magnets drawing your fingers together closer and closer, more and more powerfully, try to resist if you must but the magnets are too powerful drawing these fingers closer and closer try to stop them, ... but the more you try the more powerful the magnet attraction becomes, closer and closer more and more powerfully,"

Continue until the fingers touch.

Here we have learned to use the *Try Effect or Principle*, there are certain things that the human mind is hard wired to do. One of them we learned in childhood then carried with us through most of the rest of our lives that is *to fail when we try*.

Having the subject try to resist something reinforces the fact that it will work. There is a whole science behind this **psychology of failure** that I will detail to some degree in the advanced section

In effect you are creating a **bind** within the subject that the harder they try to resist the more they will fail.

The phrase is often used by hypnotists like this ***"try not to relax as you sit in this really comfortable chair"***. Or *"try not to focus on my voice as I speak"*

Phrases such as these are very powerful, because as the subject tries not to, they are actually focusing more.

This convincer is a good starting point to introduce the WOW factor for instant hypnosis techniques. Later we are going to revisit this suggestibility test as an induction, as way of creating instant hypnosis effects that is so simple yet so effective that you may be surprised.

THE HAND GRASPING TEST

This suggestibility test is known by several names Hands Locked, Interlocking Fingers along with a few others. The hands are closed together, fingers interlaced, the subject is unable to get his or her hands apart.

Personally I have always tended to shy away from this test; it was in the early days of my journey into hypnosis, a difficult one for me to do. Possibly because it was the first test I ever did on anyone ... it failed.

Later as I became more creative, understood what was happening I became very good at inducing the effect, The point is, don't give up, persevere, hypnosis is about confidence, if you are confident as a hypnotist then your subject will believe in you, apply the underlying principles and you will be successful.

Once again sit your subject down facing you, take their hands have then raise their arms to about chest height, interlock the fingers, now take their hands in yours, say the following

" just imagine that right now your hands are becoming stuck fast , clued together, tighter and tighter, (squeeze their hand as you say this to demonstrate how tight they are becoming, and of course to install your anchor for later use)

Those fingers are becoming clued tight locked together so tight that you won't be able to open them squeeze them now tighter and tighter so tight that the knuckles turn white, and now I'm placing clue all over them, so that they are locked even tighter sealed and you won't be able to open them it's as if I'm pouring super clue, industrial strength all over them, and on top of that I'm sealing them in cement quick drying cement that won't allow you to get your hands apart it's too tight as you squeeze your fingers so tight so hard that it will be impossible for you to separate your hands, the harder you try the stronger the clue and cement becomes sealing those hands tighter ,, until I tell you it's OK to let them apart. Clued tightly now,, keep squeezing them together tighter and tighter, so when I count to three, you will try to get your hands apart, but you won't be able to, the clue will become stronger and tighter sticking your hands together the more you struggle the tighter and more solidly stuck tighter your hands will become,,, 1, 2, 3, try now but you won't be able to get them apart,"

By now you should recognise the **Anchoring Stages** the **Command Stages, Disassociation Stages**, the **Descriptive Wording** plus many of the other subtleties in this convincer

For those that may have missed it here are the stages presented in this convincer

Those fingers (disassociation) are becoming ***clued tight locked together*** (Descriptive Wording)so tight that you won't be able to open them ***squeeze them now tighter and tighter*** (commanding the subject to squeeze their hands together) ***so tight that the knuckles turn white***, and ***now I'm placing clue all over them,*** (descriptive wording) so that they are locked even tighter sealed ***and you won't be able to open them*** (commanding the subject) it's ***as if*** (the as if technique) I'm pouring ***super clue, industrial strength*** (descriptive wording)all over them, and on top of that I'm sealing them in cement quick drying cement ***that won't allow you to get your hands apart*** (commanding the subject) it's too tight as ***you squeeze your fingers so tight so hard that it will be impossible for you to separate your hands,*** (commanding the subject) ***the harder you try the stronger the clue and cement becomes*** (single bind) sealing those hands tighter ,, ***until I tell you it's OK*** to let them apart. (Commanding the subject) Clued tightly now,, keep squeezing them together tighter and tighter, (commanding the subject) so when I count to three, ***you will try to get your hands apart, but you won't be able to,*** (commanding the subject) the clue will become stronger and tighter sticking your hands together the more you struggle the tighter and more solidly stuck tighter your hands will become,,, 1, 2,

3, *try now but you won't be able to get them apart,*" (commanding the subject)

The skill is to deliver each of these key phrases in such a way as they appear to be normal conversation. Beyond this all I can say is practise be creative.

THE HYPNOTIC ITCH
CHC TESTING, NON-AWARENESS SETS OR MIND FU*K LEVEL ONE

CHC stands for *Covert Hypnotic Command*, before we leave the subject of convincers or tests I want to introduce you to a very powerful technique for testing a subject without their conscious awareness.

Most hypnotic states occur naturally or outside our awareness, if you've ever watched somebody deeply intent on a television show you will see them nodding in agreement with the points of a show or throwing their hands up or getting upset when they disagree with something in the show. During a movie they will glaze over leaning forward as if to get closer to the screen getting more into the plot. These physical reactions are unconscious people don't know they are doing them. It is similar to not realising you are tapping your foot to music, or checking your phone every five minutes people are reacting subconsciously to some outside stimuli.

Another example of this is that friend of ours (*we all know this guy*) who always picks up the cigarette lighter placing it in his pocket, claiming unconscious ownership of the lighter. Indeed he already had four others there, he is performing unconscious physical reactions, he is in a mild state of hypnotic trance he will remain partially unaware of what he is doing

Most of the time we are in fact in a light trance state, the body is following along with whatever seems like reasonable suggestions.

Next time you want to test a person for suggestibility yet you don't want them to be exactly aware of the test, apply the principles you have learned above, start telling them a story, a story that involves a physical reaction, like the itch story.

"you know what I hate I hate it when you get those undefined tingles that turns into an itch, the itch that niggles at your skin till you can't help but scratch it, it's always at a different place on your body, it just starts,, out of nowhere and next thing you know your scratching and that scratching feels really good because it relieves the itch"

Paraphrase this into your own words, creating a story a compelling story about the sensation of itching, anyone hearing it will feel that itch perhaps even be compelled to have a good deep scratch, it may be brief almost a throw away action, or it may come a few minutes after the story. Conversely you might also notice that people who overhear the story are scratching.

Also try this, simply state that you are thirsty, that you could do with a drink, the first person who says **yeah me too**, is possibly susceptible to hypnosis. (Or thirsty as well)

There is of course no reason this psychological effect cannot be used to create erotic effects. As long as you are descriptive, delivering the information in the right way at the right time. (*Timing is an art form in itself as you don't want to seem like a creep when you start using sexual language*) descriptions and words are powerful things, did you know for example that there are people who get turned on just by reading the descriptions of the porn they are about to watch. The wording used to describe what they are going to see alone is enough to start the physiological reactions firing anchors or triggers.

Advertisers have known this for years, good copyrighters will appeal to the emotions of their readers making them want products they don't really need.

So what started as an experiment with an itch or making someone feel thirsty can be applied to your testing in erotic hypnosis, simply by talking to someone in the right way can reveal a lot about whether or not they are a good candidate for hypnosis at all.

But *what* to say with *when* to say it are the key factors here. This is where research and getting as much information as possible can help you.

Let's assume you are trying to instil a sexual idea in the mind of your subject. Taking into account that you may already be in a relationship that lends itself to this type of thing. Then the information that most woman take into account the **location** in their fantasies would be of great benefit. Did you know that recent research reveals that some 82 percent of both men and women have sexual fantasies that involve or are centred around an unusual location, an out of the ordinary spot?

You might for example start talking about locations that you know your subject has already fantasied about. This way you don't have to mention sex at all. Handling this in the right way can change your outcomes tremendously.

By now you should have a clear idea of what's involved, how to do the suggestibility tests or convincers. There are many more that I will detail in the later sections of this work, for the moment remember you are looking for compliance, you are convincing the subject that hypnosis is possible for them, you are also demonstrating that you have learned the skills which lay behind the techniques and the principles of hypnosis, in the meantime practise and enjoy

In time you are going to easily apply principle of storytelling to your suggestibility tests. Once you get creative allowing your imagination to express itself. Adding the element of storytelling or expressive language to your work as a hypnotist will enable you to experiment with different ideas during these tests.

WAKING HYPNOSIS

There is a lot of conjecture as to whether or not the state of being wide awake while hypnotised (***Waking or Covert Hypnosis)*** is possible. It's not the kind of thing we can actually do research on, as it is somewhat vague in its nature. The evidence relies for the most part on anecdotal evidence. That anecdotal evidence however is remarkably strong, even compelling.

Dave Elman tells the story of how his son hated dentists, specifically needles. Elman went through an elaborate ruse involving the delivery of a magic medicine that stopped the pain of needles. To cut a long story short his son behaved as if the medicine were real. You will know this as the placebo effect.

Elman's son acted much as you would expect of a hypnotised subject, who had been given the post hypnotic suggestion, that the medicine would take away the pain of a needle. The point being that no hypnotic process occurred. Creating this effect on a child who trusts you as a parent is one thing, but not proof.

Derren Brown performs an effect where he tells a medical student that by simply stoking the side of his jaw three times, he will induce a tooth ache similarly I've created complete anaesthesia with the same process.

I'm sure we have all, at some point in our flippant youth, convinced a room full of people that there is a bad smell in the air, if you haven't, then you should try it, walk into a room screw up your nose, sniff the air exclaiming ...***"my god,,, what's that terrible smell***". People will begin to smell it as well, or believe they can, based partly on the power of your acting, partly on the fact that they weren't expecting it, they have no ***Conscious Evidence*** to the contrary the effect also works partly because you are Inducing ***Olfactory Hallucination.***

If you find someone really well dressed who had clearly spent hours getting ready, ask them to "***turn around, Ok turn around the*** *other way. **Ok I know what's wrong with that now**"* simply walk away. It's a cruel trick but a very good demonstration of the power of suggestion or **Implied Information**. As they will spend the rest of the day worrying about what's wrong, even when several people check for them telling them everything is Ok, they will still get three or more people to double check.

So what has this to do with erotic hypnosis? Actually a lot, with a little practise you can induce hypnotic states in a subject simply by saying something in the right way. Language is a very powerful thing.

If we look at what happened in our example of telling someone that something was wrong with their cloths, we are actually creating a situation where that person has **substituted** their own **Critical Analysis** for yours, in fact this can be so powerful if done properly that the subject will feel uneasy right up until they change their cloths altogether.

Another example of the power of this substitution is, arriving at the dentist's office bent over in a screaming ball of pain, only to have the pain begin fading away as you walk up to the receptionists desk.

The dominant submissive relationship is already predisposed to this type of effect. For example did you know that it is now a proven fact that some seventy per cent of people, vanilla or otherwise will react to an authority figure in a certain predictable way. Did you know that we all have auditory hallucinations, which a good hypnotist can utilise, ask ten people if they have ever heard their name called when there was no one around, at least five will say they have. The principle is now being taught to doctors in emergency rooms. An accident victim arrives all busted up, while laying down the hapless victim catches the words *"nothing serious, he'll survive"* the patient starts picking up immediately showing signs of improvement. Because we have a **pre- frame** about things said by authority figures.

On the dark side of this is the Nuremburg Defence where many of the Nazis said as a defence (read excuse) "I was just following orders" it turns out they were, just following orders, to the point where they would do things, that had you asked them before the war, they would have claimed they would never do.

AUTHORITY SHIFT

An effective hypnosis technique called the *Authority Shift* which if performed successfully can create instant compliance then hypnosis, here's how to do it...

Let's assume your partner has a problem, the problem itself is not as important as the technique I am going to teach here, it is as always the principle that is important, how you do this is up to you, actually I'd be interested to hear any clever applications of this effect

To keep it simple I will explain the technique using the "gag reflex" Not the first thing you thought of... During any medical examination that involves the throat, when the uvula is touched it causes a natural gagging response.

Now you could spend weeks of practise or training to overcome it. Or you could place your subject in a trance state, then include as part of your script something that goes along these lines

"Now I'm giving you a pencil whenever you're holding this pencil you will easily be able to override your natural gag response, your gag reflex is perfectly natural, its nature's way of protecting you, but it can be easily controlled and over ridden, just as breathing is natural, yet you can hold your breath... controlling that natural response, because breathing is something you don't think about... you just do... naturally... so as you hold this pencil and as you feel it in your hand you won't gag ... its easily and effective ...you will find you can't gag as long as you're holding this pencil. That's all there is to it, just hold onto the pencil and you will actually enjoy it,"

Notice that we didn't try to deny that there is a gagging response we used it, making it part of our other natural responses although short (it should really be part of your larger scripting) it uses an authority shift, along with other techniques I will explain at a later date... make it your own add to it bend it utilize it, enjoy it. As you may have guessed this is only an example it would be a little silly to have someone rushing off to find a pencil during certain activities.

When creating hypnotic effects keep in mind that sex isn't just one thing. Many newbies rush in, getting to the hard stuff much too quickly. Focus on the pre as well as the after effects, Sex is about sensual pleasure. Enjoyment. Excitement. Ecstasy.

The thrill of physically touching, being touched by another warm body, the rising excitement toward sexual release, the climactic ecstasy of orgasm. The pulsating, afterglow of relaxation following orgasm *implies* that the act has already occurred, that it was enjoyable.

As we discussed implication is much more powerful than direct statements. Keep in mind as you create your *hypnotic itches* that sexuality also serves both a psychological and spiritual purpose.

Later we will examine how to use this technique with a few others for all kinds of effects, from enjoying a certain smell, taste or sensation, to being more creative in and out of the bedroom.

Here are two ways of looking at or dealing with authority shifts. Firstly in the world of erotic hypnosis, it might describe, as the submissive, slave or bottom (choose your own terminology) handing over authority to the Hypnotist, Master, Owner, Sir (once again choose your own description).

The second is where the authority for a claim or suggestion comes from an outside source which carries with it a certain amount of believable authority. For example some people are more prone to believe things they read in the newspaper or see on TV.

Claiming something is normal or natural carries more authority or becomes believable if everybody else is doing it. There's an old advertising ploy that goes like this. *More People Enjoy Product X Than Ever Before.* Or *Join Hundreds of Others in Your Area by Using Product Z*

The premise being that everybody else is doing it, so this makes it OK even necessary for you to do it as well. As you are constructing your hypnotic influences, tests, inductions or scripting you might want to keep this in mind.

LANGUAGE MODALS

There are three ways people receive authority messages. There are also two input methods.

Let me explain...

Humans tend to receive information about the world through their ***Representational System***. Either ***Sight, Sound*** or ***Auditory and Kinaesthetically***. If you know which of these your subject's **Prime Modality** is, it becomes much easier to input the information directly into your subject's subconscious mind. To bypass the critical analytical part of the brain.

People are more accepting of information that complies or agrees with how they see the world. Some people see the world visually others through what they hear, still others through touch or direct contact with their environment. In reality we all have a mixture or soup of modalities, yet one is always more prominent that the others.

NLP Neuro-Linguistic Programming teaches us that in most circumstances people, will have four sensory based modes directing their day-to-day mental processing, these are...

Visual cues - sight, mental imagery, spatial awareness

Auditory cues - sound, speech, dialog (linguistic)

Kinaesthetic sense - somatic feelings in the body, temperature, pressure, and emotion.

Digital- thoughts, internal dialogue

The other two senses, gustatory (taste), olfactory (smell), have more to do with activating the memory. Which are dealt with separately. As we progress this knowledge with its application will become invaluable to you

For example, as a hypnotist especially an erotic hypnotist, part of your craft will involve creating **Feedback Loops**

A feedback loop is where you have the subject feel something, describe it to you, you in turn tell them what to feel next by using the language they just used to describe it.

For example there are several way to describe almost anything. The weather, bloody hot, too cold just right.

Ask someone what the weather is going to be like tomorrow. Listen to their language as they describe it, listen to how they feel about it or what their plans are.

Tune into key words, you're looking for words that describe their personal modality words that describe vision, seeing, looking are visual keys.

Hearing, listening sound words are auditory keys

While touch feel sense words are Kinaesthetic. For example, a person might say the weather *looks* good today, or it *feels* like it might rain. A feedback loop is created as you feed their own primary language back to them later. Have you ever *looked* at hypnosis, have you ever wondered what it *feels* like to be hypnotised.

By listening carefully to the way people use words you'll be able to pick up on their primary language model. *I've **seen** movies about it, I've **heard** this before, I've **read** a book on this, don't know I've never **thought** about it, gosh that shirt is a bit **loud**.*

During the various stages of hypnosis, you will feedback their own language to them as a normal part of your speech patterns, phrases such as

*Maybe you **feel** more **comfortable** as you relax, have you ever **seen** a person truly relaxed, you know what it **looks like**, **listen** to your own breathing now as you relax more and more deeply, just **pay attention** to the **natural rhythms** of your body.*

Very quickly this type of speech will become very natural for you, a good way to practise is to use this to build rapport with everybody you speak to. It's a great way to build unconscious connections with people as everybody tends to listen to themselves.

INDUCTIONS

It is now time to move onto the fabulously wonderful world of hypnotic inductions. The art of actually getting your subject into state. There are few things more rewarding than achieving your first true deep hypnosis, having the subject return to the waking state, saying hey that was really cool do it again.

Ok there are some physical things that surpass it, mountain climbing, combative arts, orgasm...but from the point of view of psychology or your journey as a hypnotist there are few greater senses of achievement.

As we examine each of these inductions I will be exploring the actual art of hypnosis as well. So make sure you read all of it, study each section, learning as you learn.

Many of these inductions can be done straight out of the convincer stage, I have always felt a little uneasy about hypnotists who separate the stages, doing a test breaking into normal conversation, then starting all over again with the hypnosis stage, if you have experience or you put in a lot of practise this it will work, However I have always found it more productive to keep the flow going to move from one state naturally into the next,

For example let's assume I am doing the eyes wide shut test, the subject can't open their eyes. For just the briefest moment I let them try, then I reach over gently tilt their head forward, as if to help them sleep, then without missing a beat I start one of the inductions.

"That's good now just relax and let go, let that relaxation in the eyes begin to spread throughout the entire body, into the muscles of the face relaxing the cheeks ... All those tiny muscles in the forehead and even those around the mouth, just above the eye brows and spreading behind the ears, relaxing deeply ... each muscle letting go relaxing deeper and sounder... letting all the muscles of the face and head become limp. Loose ... going deeper now"

Wherever possible you should try to create this natural flow,

SOME IMPORTANT RECAPS

Wherever possible alter these induction scripts to fit the prime language of your subject, listen carefully to how they use language, then use that same language , feeding it back to them, *not the exact same words but the language.*

Hypnosis is not sleep, if your subject falls asleep then starts snoring, you have done something wrong. In therapy hypnosis is used to learn, to create new patterns of thought, new ways of doing things, removing old habits, replacing them with good new habits.

Learning is active; we must be consciously involved in the process of learning. The mind needs to pay attention, absorb the information, this is also true of erotic hypnosis, for your commands to be effective, be they direct, hidden or post hypnotic, the subject must be awake, in short, they should be aware of those suggestions.

Yes, even though at first it appears that you are directing the subject toward sleep, by using language such as *Sleep Deep Now* you are actually directing them toward a state of hypnotic sleep not normal sleep

Hypnosis is a state of **Ultra-Awareness**, where the subject is focused only on you the hypnotist. Aware of what you're suggesting, compliant to those suggestions. To create this state we use various inductions, different inductions will more readily apply to different situations; realistically however you could use any induction in any situation.

WATCH THE WATCH

This is possibly the best known of all hypnotic inductions even today with advances in psychology and language patterns this is still an old favourite. However nobody is going to watch a watch, the method we are using is actually called **The Fixation Method**, so technically it could be a watch, a pen, a ring or any other object that the subject becomes fixated on, (ok if you want to go all traditional then use an old fob watch) or have the subject stare at a point on the wall, just above eye level.

Another well-known variation of this is the hypnotic spiral, although slightly different the principle method is the same, the subject becomes intently focused on the hypnotic spiral. If it is spinning we employ a different technique known as a **Reality Shift** which I will detail later.

In workshops I teach these inductions first as parts are self-working, making it easier for the beginning hypnotist.

When the human mind becomes fixated on something, such as a TV show, a book, your hypnotic spinning disk or some activity, it tends to block every other thing out, this filtering process can be used to create the hypnotic state, because the subject is already half way there.

Have the subject comfortable, sitting in a chair or lying down, keeping in mind that later you may ask them to do certain things so think ahead on this one.

Have your subject direct their gaze at the **fixation object** watch pen etc. they should not shift their focus.

Now say the following

*"Now just focus on this pen for me, Stare at it. (*Hold the pen or whatever it is just above eye level, so that the subject must strain the eyes ever so slightly to look at it, this causes eye fatigue*) Fix your eyes on it. Now take a deep breath. Hold it for a moment, now let it go just release the air from your lungs ... and feel that relaxation in the shoulders... (*They should actually feel relaxed in the shoulders as they drop with the outward breath*) now Just keep breathing deeply. Listening to the sound of my voice... now you will find that those eyelids are starting to get heavy. Very heavy and relaxed Almost as if they have heavy weights attached to them, and the more you focus on the pen the more your eyelids get heavy, tired very heavy and tired almost as if they are drawn down by those weights, of their*

own volition, heavy, very tired and heavier still you may even find that you begin to blink (if they do blink say this line immediately after) *and you blink, it becomes harder to keep them open and they have a feeling like something is pulling them down, shutting down ... like heavy curtains in a dark room, sleepy relaxed and just closing down... heavier and heavier as if they wanted to slowly close, all by themselves because they are so heavy and tired and they just want to relax, the effort of keeping them open become too much, in fact all you can think about right now is how good it will feel to just let them close and release the pressure of trying to keep them open,... getting drowsier and sleepier and heavier. And you have a feeling as if they are... slowly closing, slowly closing, getting drowsier and more tired, and when they finally do close... you know how good you'll feel. Drowsy, wonderfully relaxed... those eyes heavy now, , pulling down, deeper, down, slowly closing, getting harder and harder to see, as the lips shut down heavy... and deeply relaxed, just as when you sleep, when you're ready for a deep sleep. And you feel good... don't you as you relax even deeper... it is Very, difficult very hard to keep the eyes open, now feel that very soon they will close tightly,... almost tightly closing, just closing now, tightly closing.*

Your eyes are tightly closed; you feel good; you feel comfortable; wonderfully relaxed and able to focus on that relaxation, directing to every part of your body deeply soundly relaxed now relaxed all over; and it's Ok to just let yourself drift and enjoy this comfortable relaxed state. You are safe and free,, nobody is expecting anything of you,,, it's safe to relax and let go... just drift deeper and deeper down into relaxation You may find that your head will get heavier; to drop forward some, (or sink back into the chair)as the relaxation moves outward, into every muscle of the body, the neck, and outward through the muscles of the face... and you just let yourself drift in an easy, calm, relaxed state" deeper now, deeper and sounder into deep sleep.

Remember from the convincer section that the three dots ... means time what you saying so the sentence after the dots is spoken *as* the subject is breathing out.

Don't worry if you don't get this right every time. As long as the majority of times you are saying the important sentence on the out breath.

You will also notice a lot of dissociation, commands and image creation in the scripting,

Those Eyes "*heavier and heavier as* if they wanted *to slowly close, all* by themselves *because* they are *so heavy and tired and* they just want *to relax*",

The implication being that the eyes are able to operate independently of the subject that the eyes are getting heavy, relaxing all by themselves. Another good pattern is *all they can think about is relaxing down and closing,* or *all those arms can think about is how comfortable it would be to just rest down on the table or your lap.* Obviously eyelids, arms feet or any body part can't think for themselves, the implication however is that they can, that they are acting operating independently of the subject.

The first line is a direct command "Now just focus on this pen for me, *Stare at it.* Even though it is delivered in a gentle even friendly tone, it will be received as a command to follow all further instructions.

We have also introduced a few new concepts that you can apply to all your hypnosis

As you re read the script you will notice that the hypnotist is giving permission to the subject to relax to let go, making it OK to release. *"You know how good you'll feel. Drowsy, wonderfully relaxed"... nobody is expecting anything of you... it's safe to relax and let go*

Plus we have added a bit of descriptive or story telling language *"they have a feeling like something is pulling them down, shutting down ... like heavy curtains in a dark room, sleepy relaxed and just closing down... heavier and heavier as if they wanted to slowly close, all by themselves because they are so heavy and tired and they just want to relax"*

This is called **layering**, where several ideas are given to the subject at the same time, where more than one meaning can be taken from a statement, you are describing a dark room, which *implies* sleep, with **focus** which implies being awake *and able to focus on that relaxation* the subjects unconscious mind doesn't know which to react to, or follow.

They will therefore do both, which places them in a trance state.

MILTON ERICKSON

This might be a good time to mention...One of the greatest influences on modern hypnotherapy Milton Erickson, he's innovations were so profound that there is a method that bears his name. I suggest if you want to study hypnosis beyond the pages of this book that you make a study of him and his work. In the short form however, Erickson had a particular way of inducing the state of hypnosis, using captivating stories and metaphor.

As we progress through the inductions in this book you will be given powerful examples of this technique.

The first principle is that something *implied* is going to be more powerful than something ***directly stated***. In the negative sense telling someone they are messy or untidy is less effective than telling them a story about another person who is messy then getting them to agree that this is a bad thing.

In a similar way ***implying sleep*** is going to be more effective than saying ***you will sleep now***,

You can intensify any induction by observing your subjects reactions, timing your suggestions very closely with those reactions. For example, the remark, ***"Occasionally, they are going to blink,"*** during a test or induction might be said immediately after you notice the subject blink.

HAND TO FACE METHOD

Somewhat advanced in appearance, yet still using the basic principles is the hand to face method

Get your subject as comfortable as possible, hands resting on the arms of a chair.

Now here's the clever bit, you are going to *train* your subject to enter the state of hypnosis, without them being fully aware that any training is going on. This is called fractionation more on this later.

This could be considered as the first way of introducing a *trigger* into your hypnotic work. We have dealt briefly with anchors, so now let's look at triggers.

By definition a trigger is used to fire anchors that you have placed within your subjects mind. A trigger can also be a sound that is used in the same way an anchor is used, so instead of touching the subject to cause a reaction an emotion or feeling, you are creating the same effect with a sound or noise. To my way of thinking, an anchor is any touch that causes emotional or state change, such as handshakes hugs kisses caresses. While a trigger is any sound that causes a state or makes the subject to do something, or perform an action. A loud bang makes us jump, the heart races or the theme music of a movie or an old song on the radio makes us revisit certain scenes or feelings we have experienced.

Hence you will notice a lot of stage hypnotists say...*And when I snap my fingers*, this causes the sound of the snap to become a trigger to obey the hypnotist.

The best known example of this is Pavlov's dogs, we all know the story when the dogs heard the sound of the bell they began salivating, expecting food. Now I'm not saying your submissive is a dog, unless they want to be (see advanced section) the trigger could be any reasonable sound, a section of music, the phone, your voice, or anything else that is appropriate to the goal or commands you have in mind.

THE INDUCTION

While this induction may seem simple or relatively straight forward there is a lot science behind it. Which we will examine at the end.

In just a moment, when I ask you to, I am going to have you bring one of your hands up in front of your eyes, just like this Demonstrate the hand position. Palm of the hand facing in towards their face, with fingers pointing upward held lightly together. The important part here is the fact that you are showing them what you want them to do. This pre-frames or trains them, in a sense to follow your commands

Now just let those eyes close and listen to my voice... (Wait for them to breathe out) *in a moment I will snap my fingers and when I do you are going to open your eyes, and pick a spot on your hand.*

You might find it difficult to open the eyes, and then hard to keep them open, which is only natural since you have been relaxing so comfortably.

I am going to want you to try, and open your eyes, and with a little effort you will be able to get them open. It will be hard, but you can open them,

Now, the one thing that you must accomplish is to remain totally relaxed I want you to, stay completely relaxed even with your eyes open, you will be completely deeply relaxed and with your hand in this position.

Remaining relaxed, and at ease, just let your hand move, up in front of your face with the fingers pointed upward, and pressed together. *Just like I showed you before*

And you will pick a spot on your hand and stare at it, I want you to focus all your attention on that spot, really concentrate on it. Bring your whole mind to it.

Now, (snap your fingers) *attempt to open your eyes, and pick one spot on your hand, and begin to concentrate on it. Focus*

(Wait for them to open the eyes repeating that even though it is difficult they can do it)

Now in a moment I'm going to snap my fingers again at that sound and as you concentrate on that one spot on your hand and one spot only, your fingers are going to spread apart. They will just gently and softly spread apart ... separating

When you hear the sound of my fingers snapping you will not have to make them spread, they will just do it themselves they will relax and just drift apart ,,,in a natural way... but do not try and stop them ... concentrate, and just allow things to take place.

(Snap)

Feel them spreading apart now. Just as they relax and find a natural position automatically separating now ... I wonder if it is beginning to feel as though there was a string tied to each finger pulling them apart, Separating, further, and further.

(Once the fingers have separated, proceed in the following way)

Now, do not let it disturb you that the drowsy, heavy feeling in your eyes is becoming stronger now that your fingers have spread apart. In fact you will probably notice that as your fingers spread apart, your eyes became really focused and intent on what you were doing, so now when I snap my fingers again, they will close, shutting down deeply closed

(Snap)

It is a very normal, natural sensation. They close and now as I to count from 10 down to 1 that heavy, drowsy feeling will continue to grow stronger.

From here you will flow into your **Deepening Technique**.

Let's have a look at a few of the things we learned and applied in this induction.

Primarily you are training or **conditioning** the subject to obey or comply when you snap your fingers, you did this in stages, stage one you introduced the idea, by demonstrating what you wanted them to do, this appears safe even easy, the subject offers no resistance because it appears to be part of the process,

I use finger snapping because it is almost expected of a hypnotist, that's not to say with a little creative rewording you could use a bell or some other sound.

In some of my larger more adult shows I have a routine called instant orgasm, where everyone on stage has the most intense orgasm they have ever experienced, if you are watching the show, you will believe that the effect is created through the medium of a glass of water, a snap of the fingers or a cough.

This however is a bit of a ruse; the glass of water is used to disguise the fact that I have conditioned the volunteers to react to a certain sound.

In stage two you are repeating the process, making it perfectly Ok even sort of natural to follow suggestions associated with a sound, ***when you hear the sound of my fingers snapping you will not have to make them spread, they will just do it themselves*** in the example the snap of the fingers.

Finally in stage three you have issued a direct command. ***So now when I snap my fingers again, they will close, shutting down deeply closed***

If you have played your part as the hypnotist well, your subject will from now on expect that if you tell them to do something then snap your fingers, they are compelled to follow the command.

I have also introduced a few more of very powerful language patterns

The **try technique** the **wondering language pattern**, the **X=Y pattern** as well as the **assumption pattern**.

ASSUMPTION PATTERNS

As you re-read the above induction you will notice there are a lot of assumptions being made by the hypnotist.

The induction seems to assume that the subject is already in some type of trance, there is no **Progressive Relaxation,** building to a point where the body and eyes are relaxed, we seem to just go straight into it, almost the first thing you say to the subject is that you are going to have trouble opening your eyes.

Assumption is a powerful thing, if you assume that it is a natural expected part of the process, behaving, acting as if this is what happens. Then your subject will assume that you know what you are doing and assume this as well.

Further you will have lead into this induction straight out of a convincer or test. Each flowing naturally into the other, For example if you used the eyes wide shut convincer the subjects eyes will already be relaxed, the subjects mind will easily connect your assumptions to the reality that they are going into hypnosis.

WONDERING LANGUAGE PATTERN

Wondering is a powerful Erickson technique, not only is it hypnotic language, it also gives you an **out**. If anything is *not happening* then it's ok because you were just wondering. On the surface however, when you state that you are wondering a certain thing, the subject will also wonder about it, then check, tuning into their body, nine times out of ten they will find what they are looking for.

For example if you stare into your subjects eyes, then after a moment say, ***ok now I'm just wondering if you can feel anything***. The subject will reason there must be something to feel, they will mentally start searching for anything that could be what you're referring to.

The simple fact that they are now searching their body, doing a quick mental scan. The subject is concentrating on themselves, they will inevitably find something. (If not you simple state, *"that's ok I was just wondering"*.)

X=Y PATTERN

This pattern is one of my favourites, because once you get a handle on it, it is a beautiful piece of B.S. that can really fuck with someone's mind. The idea is that one thing can be made to equal another, even against common sense.

For example in the above induction ... ***Now, do not let it disturb you that the drowsy, heavy feeling in your eyes is becoming stronger now that your fingers have spread apart. In fact you will probably notice that as your fingers spread apart, your eyes became really focused and intent on what you were doing,***

If you really think about it this doesn't make any sense, there is no reason why spreading your fingers should make your eyes heavier. Another way of expressing the X=Y pattern is to say

The More You, the Less You,

The More You, the More You.

The more you listen to my voice the less you want to keep your eyes open.

The more you focus on that spot the more your eyes become tired and heavy.

The analytical critical part of the subjects mind is bypassed by such statements as they appear perfectly reasonable they make sense, even when they don't.

For example you might say to someone, ***the more you read the better you become***. This is actually a fallacy yet it makes sense when we hear it.

There are several very good ways to use these pattern, many will be examined as we progress.

PROGRESSIVE RELAXATION INDUCTION

As you discover more about hypnosis, practise language patterns and gain experience you are going to develop your own style. Your own ways of speaking of inducing the hypnotic state,

One of the first things you are most likely to do is create your own progressive relaxation induction.

Partly because it's easy, all the subject does is sit or lay back while listening. Plus it's a very good way for you to practise.

I am going to detail one of my PRI's with the working behind it, this is a very good way to learn to **pre-frame** your subject for the erotic content you will introduce later. You are going to subtly introduce ideas and concepts during the hypnotic induction that relate to what you want to achieve as a goal for the session.

In my clinical work a client may be dealing with stress issues or self-discipline problems.

My induction, indeed even the convincer or testing stage, takes this into account, during the process I will begin inserting ideas that relate to the larger script I'm going to introduce later

For example I may in the induction say, *and notice that the stress is drifting away as you relax deeper.* The implication becomes meaningful when later I say *and notice whenever you clench and then relax your fist the stress just drifts away.*

Or in the case of self-discipline or goal setting I may casually say, *and because you know you can relax and achieve this goal, the goal of relaxing...deeply.* Later during the scripting stage I might say ... *you can relax and achieve this gaol, the goal of success or whatever you set your mind to.*

These are almost throw away lines from my point of view, but remember everything you say, goes into the subconscious at some level.

A good example of how you might alter or adapt your induction is smoking. A client comes into my office to give up smoking, I use a normal induction (after the test, before the deepener,) all three contain references that I want the client to understand at the hypnotic level. Phrases such as *you don't need any help to relax you are able to do this all by yourself*, the implication becomes apparent later during the scripting, when I say *and you don't need any help to let go of smoking you can do it all by yourself.*

So we are going to examine the PRI later you will adapt it to the erotic hypnosis work you intent to do with *your* subject.

There will be two versions of this induction the vanilla and the erotic

THE VANILLA VERSION

Have your subject sit or lay down comfortably.

Once they have settled commence as follows.

Ok just relax and close those eyes, just letting them close... now listen to my voice, paying attention to what I'm saying focus on my words ... and as you do you may feel parts of your body beginning to relax I'm not sure which parts but I do know that parts of you will relax very deeply as I talk,

So I want you to focus now on your breathing... (wait for two or three breaths) *you will notice that your breathing has changed now, it's become the type of breathing you have when you are deeply relaxing, ...and ready for sleep... the kind of sleep that's is healing ... just become aware of it, and as you focus on your breathing ...as you pay attention to it, I wonder if you notice you are relaxing , in fact does focusing on your breathing help you to relax even more deeply , soundly ... relaxing now.*

As you let your subconsciousness show you how easily you can relax, you may find yourself just letting go of worry and stress as well, and take in peace and tranquillity; if you do, want this relaxation and I believe that you do, then all you have to do is take another deep, deep breath, ... and as you exhale, just let your worries melt into that breath, so that as you exhale, those concerns, fears and anxieties will simply flow out with that breath and be gone, leaving you relaxed and comfortable

That's good you're doing really well... now just focus on the sounds around us... the sounds in this room, the sound of the traffic outside ... become aware of those sounds, in your imagination can you control those sounds ...can you make them louder as you focus on them more, can you make them more clear ... can you notice them more... and I'm just wondering if as you use your imagination to make them increase in volume... does that help you to relax even more... more deeply, soundly...

And because you are controlling your awareness of those sounds can you make them quieter...softer... can you... you use your imagination to make those sounds ...far away... soft and quite... And I'm wondering does this make you relax even more... more deeply soundly relaxed...

You notice now that all the muscles in your head are letting go and relaxing deeply, from the forehead... those muscles above the eyebrows all the way down the face, the cheek bones...even those tiny little muscles around the mouth are letting go and relaxing deeply letting go of tension anxiety and just relaxing deeply, you might notice a feeling of heaviness now spreading down from the face into the neck and shoulders. Down deeper and deeper more and more relaxed each breath that you take going deeper and deeper more soundly relaxed.

as your body and mind accept this relaxation, allowing it to happen...to occur naturally, letting go of those feelings of stress and worry, fear anxiety and relaxing even more deeply ...soundly, as you relax even more deeply heavier than you have even been before it's comfortable for you, your subconscious mind already knows how to do this, and as you relax and focus, and listen letting go of stress and worry and letting yourself more fully relax and listen to my words and with each of my words you go deeper and sounder,...deeper ... sounder

Each breath helping you to relax more and more deeply, soundly, as that relaxation and heaviness seeps down into the arms, like a liquid, flowing down heavy... through the tops of the arms ,,,the elbows into the wrists and the hands heavy and relaxed ...even to the very fingertips...

And flowing now... through the entire body making you more and more relaxed... heavier, more serene calmer and tranquil... the whole body seems to relax and grow heavier and heavier you can feel the weight of you torso... the chest and tummy getting so heavy now... so heavy that you just don't want to move... just relax and rest. And its ok to rest, because right now you are free to rest and relax... no one is expecting anything of you,,, all your troubles can just drift away... this is your time of freedom and space a time and place when you can relax and let go of any and all fears anxieties and worries,, nothing concerns you now... in fact all you can think about is how comfortable you are and how nice it would be to just... drift down ... into a deep sleep... deeply soundly asleep...

Feel how heavy those legs are as they rest there... just like heavy lead weights... the thighs taking in that liquid flow of deep relaxation... through the calves and all the way down to the tips of the toes... heavy deeply soundly relaxed.

Its ok to relax and let your worries go... it feels good to relax and the more deeply you relax the better it feels, just that feeling of being so heavy and relaxed that nothing else matters does it...

So relax deeply now ... deeply and soundly and go deeper... deeper with each word I say... with each sound that you hear, deeper sounder...

And relax

Before moving on to the erotic version let's take a moment to examine all the intricacies used in this induction, because by knowing them, you will be able to adapt your erotic inductions a lot more successfully. Each of the applications has been mentioned before however this is the first time we have used them all in the same place or as part of the overall process.

Ok just relax and close those eyes, commanding even though it is delivered in a friendly tone it should be a direction to do as you are instructed.

Just letting them close... not quite an instruction more of a direction ... giving the eyes permission to work by themselves. In fact you can add this exact phrase in as we will see in the erotic induction. Later you will be asking the subject to allow their body and feelings to work independently of them, to release themselves to whatever feelings come to them. Those feelings work alone, without the conscious awareness of the subject any effort made to deny them or hold them back will be pointless.

now listen to my voice, paying attention to what I'm saying focus on my words and as you do you may feel parts of your body beginning to relax I'm not sure which parts but I do know that parts of you will relax very deeply as I talk,

A command *listen to my voice* that is softened by the next phrase. As you do this you will relax. This is an X=Y pattern, listening to someone's voice does not mean you will automatically relax. However it makes sense in the atmosphere of hypnosis. Then we cause the subject to internalise their feelings, to focus concentrating on themselves to examine what they are feeling. ***Because there is a part of you that is relaxing. I don't know where it is, so you must go looking for it.*** Invariably the subject will find such a place simply because they are focusing on themselves. This will convince them that they are indeed relaxing. If they are relaxing just like you said, then they will reason unconsciously that they must be going into hypnosis, just like you said.

so I want you to focus now on your breathing... you will notice that your breathing has changed now, it's become the type of breathing you have when you are deeply relaxing, ...and ready for sleep... the kind of sleep that's is healing ... just become aware of it, and as you focus on your breathing ...as you pay attention to it, I wonder if you notice you are relaxing, in fact does focusing on your breathing help you to relax even more deeply , soundly relaxing now.

Distraction, you are now directing where and how the subject is thinking. The more you focus on something the more you become aware of it, the more inclined you are to notice changes in it. Those changes can actually be directed by the hypnotist.

As you let your subconsciousness show you how easily you can relax, you may find yourself just letting go of worry and stress as well, and take in peace and tranquillity; if you do, want this relaxation and I believe that you do then all you have to do is take another deep, deep breath, ...and as you exhale, just let your worries melt into that breath, so that as you exhale, those concerns, fears and anxieties will simply flow out with that breath and be gone, leaving you relaxed and comfortable

That's good you're doing really well... now just focus on the sounds around us... the sounds in this room, the sound of the traffic outside become aware of those sounds, in your imagination can you control those sounds ...can you make them louder as you focus on them more, can you make them more clear can you notice them more... and I'm just wondering if as you use your imagination to make them increase in volume,, does that help you to relax even more... more deeply, soundly...

And because you are controlling your awareness of those sounds can you make them quieter...softer... can you... you use your imagination to make those sounds ...far away... soft and quite...

just drift away... this is your time of freedom and space a time and place when you can relax and let go of any and all fears anxieties and worries,, nothing concerns you now... in fact all you can think about is how comfortable you are and how nice it would be to just... drift down ... into a deep sleep... deeply soundly asleep...

Feel how heavy those legs are as they rest there... just like heavy lead weights... the thighs taking in that liquid flow of deep relaxation... through the calves and all the way down to the tips of the toes... heavy deeply soundly relaxed.

Its ok to relax and let your worries go... it feels good to relax and the more deeply you relax the better it feels, just that feeling of being so heavy and relaxed that nothing else matters does it...

So relax deeply now ... deeply and soundly and go deeper... deeper with each word I say... with each sound that you hear... deeper sounder and relax

THE EROTIC VERSION

The ***PRI*** for Erotic Hypnosis

The following induction is virtually the same as the one above, it is a ***progressive relaxation induction***; however this time we have adapted it ever so slightly to incorporate many of the principles we have learned thus far, we will be implementing the idea of erotic control into the subjects mind.

A word of warning, make sure you have the subjects full agreement when doing this, some of these techniques and principles if applied in the right way are very powerful they might even be used without any induction, on unsuspecting members of the public. ***In our craft this is forbidden***

PROGRESSIVE RELAXATION INDUCTION

"You can enter trance now or you can try to keep your eyes open for a little longer while that delightful sense of comfort continues to fill your body? ... Ok just relax and close those eyes, just letting them close... as if giving the eyes permission to work by themselves.

To shut down of their own volition, just as your body can work by itself. now listen to my voice, paying attention to everything I'm saying, just focus on my words... and the sound of my voice and as you do,,, you may feel parts of your body beginning to relax and let go,,, I'm not sure which part will relax first, but I do know that a part of you will relax,, very deeply as I talk, just let your mind find that part, the part that is relaxing,,, now and you know it's good to relax don't you, in fact Every time you accept one of my suggestions as you are now, you will find that you relax even more, and your body will feel more relaxation comfort and serene simply because you have accepted my suggestion to relax it; and that is a good feeling isn't it... it's a wonderful way to feel...

So now I want you to focus on your breathing... just become aware of it. And as you become more aware of it, you will notice that your breathing has changed now, it's become the type of breathing you have when you are deeply relaxed, ...and ready for sleep... the kind of sleep that is healing ... energizing,,, just become aware of it, and as you focus on your breathing ...as you pay attention to it, I wonder if you notice you are relaxing ,even more in fact does focusing on your breathing helping you to relax even more deeply , soundly... relaxing now, even more deeply and soundly...

As you let your subconsciousness show you how easily you can submit yourself to deep relaxation how easy it is to let it go stress, and accept relaxation,,, you may find yourself surrendering worry as well, and you will find your mind and body accepting comfort, if you want this perfect sensation and if you want it to grow stronger,,, all you need to do is take another deep, deep breath,... and as you exhale, let your subconsciousness mind calm your worries into that breath, so that as you exhale, those worries will simply escape with that breath and melt away, leaving you heavy,,, more relaxed deeply ,,,soundly relaxed

You already know that, your subconsciousness mind is fully aware of everything that goes on around you, and so when you're ready, just let your consciousness surrender, letting go all those things that hold you back from the pleasure , comfort , relaxation you deserve to feel,

... you deserve, and naturally want these feelings perhaps there is part of you that even needs these sensations... it perfectly natural and normal to want to feel good ...it is perfectly normal to receive pleasure, so that the more you relax and let go,, the more powerful those positive feelings, that pleasure, can become, and because this is what you want, isn't it, it's very easy to submit to those feelings it becomes easier and easier to give in to those amazing feelings, so they can grow and grow inside you, isn't that right?... yes

That's good you're doing really well... now just focus on the sounds around us... paying attention to them ... the sounds in this room ... the sound of the traffic outside become aware of those sounds, in your imagination can you control those sounds ...can you make them louder as you focus on them more... can you make them more clearer can you notice them more... and I'm just wondering if, as you use your imagination to make them increase in volume,, does that help you to relax even more... more deeply soundly...

and as you do this as you focus on those sounds all the thoughts, the worries, the stress, that make you resist those feelings of pleasure and joy can just melt away, as your subconsciousness helps you release them And because you are controlling your awareness of those sounds, can you now make them quieter...softer... can you?... you use your imagination to make those sounds ...far away... soft and quite.. And I'm wondering does this make you relax even more... more deeply soundly relaxed...so that you can enjoy all those positive feelings you asked for, and the more you surrender those resistances, the more room there will be inside you for pleasure, comfort and relaxation, which everyone wants,

so as you surrender to yourself to those feelings of pleasure and comfort and relaxation as you let go to that feeling of deep heaviness, you notice now that all the muscles in your head are letting go and relaxing deeply, moving down ,,,from the forehead... those muscles above the eyebrows all the way down the face, the cheek bones...even those tiny little muscles around the mouth are letting go and relaxing deeply... letting go of tension anxiety and just relaxing deeply, you might notice a feeling of heaviness now spreading down from the face into the neck and shoulders.

it's perfectly natural to want those feelings of pleasure... and for feelings of tranquillity and thoughtlessness to get stronger, it's perfectly normal and natural to enjoy those feelings more deeply , so that the more you relax and let go the more your conscious mind surrenders, and the more your subconsciousness opens itself, and as your mind opens to these feelings and sensations the more you yourself are open to them , to those pleasing feelings,,, go down now, Down deeper and deeper more and more relaxed each breath that you take going deeper and deeper more soundly relaxed. Creating more and more pleasure...

as your body and mind accept this relaxation and comfort, allowing it to just happen very naturally, because it is natural isn't it, to feel good and comfortable and relaxed ,,your subconsciousness can accept the freedom, of letting go, letting go of feelings of stress and worry, fear anxiety and relax even more deeply ...soundly, and there is nothing for you to do now, there is no stress,,, no worry nothing for you to do, no one is expecting anything of you ,, this is your time to just let go and surrender to the relaxation your time to surrender to those wonderful feelings that are growing in you now. and you don't even have to help your conscious mind to focus on my words, all you have to do is... relax and enjoy the sensations of relief, relaxation, and comfort and the pleasure this gives you as you relax even more deeply... just allow it to occur all by itself,,, becoming heavier than you have even been before it's comfortable for you, your subconscious mind can do all this, and as you relax and focus, and listens each word brings you relaxation and pleasure... letting go of stress and worry and letting yourself more fully relax and listen to my words... with each of my words you go deeper and sounder,...deeper ... sounder

Each breath helping you to relax more and more deeply,,, soundly, as that relaxation and heaviness seeps down into the arms, like a liquid, flowing down heavy... through the tops of the arms ,,,the elbows into the wrists and the hands heavy and relaxed ...even to the very fingertips... As you let my words into your mind, you can learn to surrender the stress inside you, and free yourself to enjoy relaxation, so if you want this, which would only be natural,,,, then let yourself ... let yourself allow it to happen,,, let yourself surrender to those feelings of relaxation pleasure and tranquillity

And that pleasure flowing now... through the entire body making you more and more relaxed... heavier, more serene calmer and tranquil... the whole body seems to relax and grow heavier and heavier you can feel the weight of your torso... the chest and tummy getting so heavy now... so heavy that you just don't want to move... just relax and rest. And its ok to rest, because right now you are free to rest and relax... free to feel as good as you want ...no one is expecting anything of you,,, all your troubles can just drift away... this is your time of freedom and space a time and place when you can relax and let go of any and all fears anxieties and worries,, nothing concerns you now... in fact all you can think about is how comfortable you are and how nice it would be to just... drift down ... into a deep sleep... deeply soundly asleep...

you might find your subconsciousness wanting to help your consciousness mind surrender, to me, this has always been a very natural thing a better way of thinking... so that all those negative thoughts that get in the way of your relaxation just drift away, far away, letting your subconscious surrender your thoughts, so that you can be filled... with deep relaxation, which is what you truly desire very deeply ...don't you

Feel how heavy those legs are as they rest there... just like heavy lead weights... the thighs taking in that liquid flow of deep relaxation... through the calves and all the way down to the tips of the toes... heavy deeply soundly relaxed.

And you already know my words are helping you to relax and let go, don't you? Some people find the idea of hypnosis... just as you are experiencing it right now... overwhelming, appealing it's as if every word I have said, or will say... takes you deeper and deeper into relaxation and pleasure, and takes you further into trance,... it is true that my words and my voice have a profoundly relaxing effect on you, because you allow them to, you allow my words to affect you deeply so that as my words relax you, you find that you can easy accept any suggestion I give you as True.

And Its ok to relax and let your worries go... it feels good to relax and the more deeply you relax the better it feels, just that feeling of being so heavy and relaxed that nothing else matters does it... and you want to relax and feel good don't you... it's a truly wonderful thing, to let go,, to surrender and relax, and this is true isn't it.

So relax deeply now ... deeply and soundly and go deeper... deeper with each word I say... with each sound that you hear, deeper sounder...

You already know each time you accept one of my suggestions, it helps you, to feel good and relax, don't you. Just like you're doing now, That my suggestions help you to surrender to those feelings, just like now, that my suggestions make you feel good… just as you do now, , and you are allowing yourself to let go… and accept, to take in my words… my voice and suggestions become more natural, Almost instinctive, existing just outside your conscious awareness. And you just naturally accept my suggestions… you accept and invite that comfort, relaxation, and pleasure more deeply each time.

And relax deeply now, more deeply than ever before…

By now you should be fully understand that there is a lot more going on here than one might first expect. That each word you say is carefully considered to affect the subject in a particular way.

That said there is no need to learn the script verbatim, it is the principles that are important.

The first idea is that you are guiding the subject into a relaxed state one body part at a time; therefore, it is important to mention each body part. This draws the attention to that part of the body following the command or suggestion to relax that section of the body.

A good tip is to move up or down the body. Starting at the head or the feet, don't jump around; this can get confusing for the subject. You will also notice new language patterns.

There are a few most you will be able to work out easily enough, but here are the important ones, with principles you will want to apply to all of your hypnosis work.

THE DOUBLE BINDING SENTENCE

The human head is an amazing thing; it contains a big meaty brain with an even more enormous mind. That mind is so clever that it can relate to more than one thing at a time, it is able to draw meaning from the smallest of clues.

Most psychic phenomena are based on this fact, that you are aware of more than you realise you are aware of. That said it can also be easily confused!

In the normal parlance a ***Double Bind*** is an emotionally distressing Catch-22 situation where an individual receives two or more conflicting messages, where one message negates the other.

This creates a situation in which the successful answer to one message results in a failed response to the other part of the message, so that the person will automatically be wrong regardless of their response. The most famous of these binds is when Groucho Marks asked "***So Tell Me Are You Still Beating Your Wife?***"

Both a yes or no answer was wrong. No means I'm not beating her now, but I used to while yes means ...yes I'm still beating my wife. It's a no-win situation.

The bind arises when the subject can't challenge the dilemma, they can't resolve it because they will look bad, without looking like they are trying to avoid the subject. They can't withdraw from the situation for exactly the same reason.

This makes double binds both difficult to respond to as well as to resist

In hypnosis double binds are used in a more positive way. As you read the script above you may have noticed it contains very carefully constructed sentences that forces the mind of your subject in the direction you want. You are using double binds to create the illusion of choice as in " "***you can ENTER TRANCE NOW or you can try to keep your eyes open for a little longer while that delightful sense of comfort continues to fill your body?*** Again this is a multi-layered technique. The command statement is presented in capitals. You would adjust your tone ever so slightly to make it a command. The illusion of choice is created between entering trance and waiting to enter trance. The outcome for the hypnotist is the same. The subject enters a trance.

"***The sounds in this room, the sound of the traffic outside become aware of those sounds, in your imagination can you control those sounds ...can you make them louder***"

LINKING PHRASES

Linking phrases are a special situation, or sentence construction where the hypnotist is actually saying two distinctly different things, while appearing to say only one thing. The subject's subconscious will react to both of them.

At first you are stating ***become aware of those sounds in your imagination*** this is an instruction to use the imagination to notice the sounds to pay attention to them. Yet at the same time the hypnotist is asking "***in your imagination can you control those sounds ...can you make them louder***"

The link is the ***in your imagination***, it creates a state where both parts of the sentence are received as one. Both meanings have influence on the subject.

As another example I have placed a few of these linking phrases or double speak commands within the script, primarily designed to introduce the erotic hypnosis concept

You might find your subconsciousness wanting to help your consciousness surrender to me this has always been a very natural process a better way of thinking...

The idea is to make this statement sound perfectly natural. Whereas in reality you are giving two distinctly different commands slipping the covert command in under the conscious radar of the subject.

The two statements are,

You might find your subconsciousness wanting to help your consciousness <u>surrender, to me</u> this has always been a very natural process a better way of thinking...

This is a clouded linking phrase, in effect your saying surrender to me, you're also saying, and it's very natural to surrender to me. About the only thing you will need to practise is the way you deliver the language pattern, there should be the slightest of unnoticed of pauses between the words ***surrender*** and ***to me***.

There are a few of them hidden in the induction a good exercise will be to find them

THE INSTANT YES SET TAG

This is possibly the oldest sales trick on the market. If you can get your customer agreeing with you a number of times he or she is likely to agree with you later, even if the thing you are asking them to agree with makes no logical sense.

Normally a yes set requires three times or points of agreement. Then the fourth is the hook. Here are a couple of examples ...

Expert sales guy: Nice day

Unsuspecting customer: Yes

Expert sales guy: I see your looking at fridges

Unsuspecting customer: Yes I am

Expert sales guy: I guess you're looking for a new fridge

Unsuspecting customer: Actually yes the old one is kaput

Expert sales guy: So I guess you like to see our new range

Unsuspecting customer: Ok yes

The idea is that the subject *falls into a pattern* of saying yes, finding themselves agreeing with the salesman.

There is a faster more effective way of achieving this yes set, we call, it **tagging**, simply by placing a tag such as *isn't it* , *won't you* or *aren't they* at the end of the statement creates a state of agreement within the subject.

So you might say something like

And you feel those muscles relax don't you,

It's better to relax isn't it?

You find yourself agreeing with me don't you?

A simple, yet highly effective technique, which we will use a lot in this next version of the induction

The above subtle changes make this a very powerful script. Don't expect to get it right the first time. Read it many times before you use it, there are many refinements within the wording that suggest things to your subject on multiple levels. Most of them you will be able to see, because you have read this whole book, followed the learning steps, you can now see between the lines.

That said here are some of the less obvious layers.

Ok just relax and close those eyes, just letting them close... **now listen to my voice, paying attention to everything I'm saying focus on my words...**

In this example we have gone from dissociation through to a direct command. In one sense the subject will dissociate themselves from the command now *listen to my voice* and obey it, because they don't see it as a command

and as you do you may feel parts of your body beginning to relax and let go I'm not sure which part will relax first but I do know that a part of you will relax,,

This causes the subject to begin looking for a part of the body that has relaxed. It is actually a command to find a part that has relaxed.

Very deeply as I talk, and it's good to relax isn't it,

This phrase is a tag it creates a sense of agreement, it makes whatever you are saying seem true even rather reasonable. After all who could reasonably dis-agree that relaxation is a good thing?

In fact Every time you accept one of my suggestions as you are now, your mind will be even more unaware that these suggestions exist, and your body will feel more relaxation comfort and serene simply because you have accepted it; and that a good feeling isn't it... it's a better way to feel...

You have probably already figured out that this next statement reinforces the yes set and creates more agreement.

you are also reinforcing the fact that the subject is accepting your suggestions **"as you are now"** is applying the **assumption** that the subject is agreeing with you doing as you ask, after all what else have they got to do while relaxing. So in effect the very fact that they are allowing you to hypnotise them means that they are also reacting to and agreeing with your suggestions.

So now I want you to focus on your breathing... just become aware of it. And as you become more aware of it, you will notice that your breathing has changed now,

This draws the subjects attention to the breathing, from this point on you will be able to control where the subject's attention is directed. As they focus on their breathing they will notice a change (*this happens every time you pay attention to your breathing there is actually nothing hypnotic about it. It is a neurological response*). Your subject will believe that the process is hypnosis, that you the hypnotist have caused this change. So from this point on, if you direct the subject to be aware of something, they will subconsciously expect some change in feelings emotions or some physical change,

It's become the type of breathing you have when you are deeply relaxing and ready for sleep... the kind of sleep that is healing ... re-energizing,

Now you are connecting the breathing to a purpose, you are telling the subject what those sensations mean.

just become aware of it, and as you focus on your breathing ...as you pay attention to it, I wonder if you notice you are relaxing, even more in fact does focusing on your breathing helping you to relax even more deeply , soundly relaxing now, even more deeply and soundly...

As you let your subconsciousness show you how easily you can surrender your stress,

STACKING: DIRECTED COMPLIANCE AND ASSUMPTION

There are many ways of stacking statements to create hidden double meanings

let it go and <u>accept</u> relaxation, you may find yourself <u>naturally</u> <u>wanting to</u> <u>surrender</u> worry as well, and accept comfort; if you do,

<u>if you want this wonderful feeling all you need to do is</u> take another deep, deep breath,…

This is a very powerful hypnotic command, it contains many layers all stacked in such a way that the subject will find it almost irresistible, finding that they are subconsciously becoming compliant. You are making it Ok to <u>surrender</u> to you, because <u>surrendering</u> to you, is good, comfortable, relaxing, even wonderful, surrendering to you creates feelings of pleasure feelings of happiness.

If you do, if you want this wonderful feeling all you need to do is take another deep,

Who wouldn't want this, this wonderful feeling, yet as you reread the statement carefully you will notice you are asking ***if you want to surrender*** because surrender now means all those good feelings.

The two things are gradually becoming intermingled in the mind of the subject, surrendering means letting go, letting go means I can relax and feel good, so to feel good I must surrender.

As you practise you will learn many ways of creating this dual state, perhaps even methods of achieving it without the need for hypnosis.

As you exhale, let your subconsciousness soothe your worries into that breath, so that as you exhale, those worries will simply escape with the breath and be gone, leaving you relaxed and comfortable

THE YOU ALREADY KNOW PRINCIPLE

Whenever you say to a subject ***you already know*** or ***your subconscious already knows***, the mind of your subject doesn't know whether or not it actually knows, so it will assume that it must know, after all why would the person hypnotising me say I know it if I didn't…

Here are a few examples…

And I'm wondering does this make you relax even more... more deeply soundly relaxed...

You notice now that all the muscles in your head are letting go and relaxing deeply, from the forehead... those muscles above the eyebrows all the way down the face, the cheek bones...even those tiny little muscles around the mouth are letting go and relaxing deeply letting go of tension anxiety and just relaxing deeply, you might notice a feeling of heaviness now spreading down from the face into the neck and shoulders. Down deeper and deeper more and more relaxed each breath that you take going deeper and deeper more soundly relaxed.

as your body and mind accept this relaxation, allowing it to happen...to occur naturally, letting go of those feelings of stress and worry, fear anxiety and relaxing even more deeply ...soundly, as you relax even more deeply heavier than you have even been before it's comfortable for you, your subconscious mind already knows how to do this, and as you relax and focus, and listen letting go of stress and worry and letting yourself more fully relax and listen to my words and with each of my words you go deeper and sounder,...deeper ... sounder

Each breath helping you to relax more and more deeply, soundly, as that relaxation and heaviness seeps down into the arms, like a liquid, flowing down heavy... through the tops of the arms ,,,the elbows into the wrists and the hands heavy and relaxed ...even to the very fingertips...

And flowing now... through the entire body making you more and more relaxed... heavier, more serene calmer and tranquil... the whole body seems to relax and grow heavier and heavier you can feel the weight of you torso... the chest and tummy getting so heavy now... so heavy that you just don't want to move... just relax and rest. And its ok to rest, because right now you are free to rest and relax... none is expecting anything of you,,, all your troubles can

In fact, your subconsciousness knows everything that goes on around you,

You already know how to act when this happens.

You already know not to lose your temper

You already know what will happen when you do this relaxation exercise.

Your subconscious already knows what makes you excited

You already know that surrendering to me is good

You already know that surrendering to your deepest desires and true self will make you feel free

This is a powerful principle that can be written into any of your scripts.

YOU ARE ALREADY READY

This technique or principle combines assumption disassociation and confusion into a single multi-level phrase

And so when it's ready, when what's ready? The subconscious, what is that? How do I know when it's ready? Perhaps it's ready now!

All this flashes through a subjects mind in less than a moment. You will notice that the subject is instantly ready once you apply this statement. Another example could be to say ***when the eyes are ready just let them close "when they are ready just let your hands drop to your lap".*** You find that people comply with this statement straight away, it's almost as if they *become* ready as soon as you make the statement.

DISCONNECTING THE SUBCONSCIOUS

Along with more disassociation, where you disconnect the eyes or the hands from the actual subject we can also dissociate the subconscious mind. Earlier we examined how making the eyes feel as if they were another far off set of eyes, made it easier to close them or lowered resistance. We can also do this with the subconscious mind. Making it easier to hand over control to the hypnotist.

You are effectively separating the subconscious from the conscious making it a 'thing', a 'thing' that at advanced levels the subject has no control over. This reinforces the idea that because the subconscious is a 'thing' it can be controlled by outside forces, in this case the hypnotist.

"It can help your consciousness surrender all those things that hold you away from the pleasure, comfort, relaxation you deserve to feel",

More reinforcement

... you deserve, and quite naturally want these feelings it perfectly natural to want to feel good ...to accept pleasure, so that the more you relax and let go the more powerful those positive feelings, that pleasure, can become, and because this is what you want anyway, it's very easy to surrender to those good feelings, so they can grow and grow inside you, isn't that right?... yes

You are connecting pleasure relaxation with compliance, they are becoming one idea, the idea that following the suggestions of the hypnotist, is actually pleasurable, later this will grow into the idea that obeying the hypnotist is natural even satisfying...

That's good you're doing really well... now just focus on the sounds around us... the sounds in this room,... the sound of the traffic outside become aware of those sounds, in your imagination can you control those sounds ...can you make them louder as you focus on them more... can you make them more clearer can you notice them more... and I'm just wondering if, as you use your imagination to make them increase in volume,, does that help you to relax even more... more deeply soundly...

And as you do this all the thoughts, the worries, the stress, that make you resist those feelings of pleasure and joy can just melt away, as your subconsciousness helps you release them

The hypnotist is now introducing a second level or layer, that resistance to the suggestions is both bad as well as unpleasant opposing or working against the suggestions will cause stress, nobody wants stress, *do they*? Resisting relaxation and pleasure is the same as resisting the suggestions, primarily those suggestions are to relax to feel good, later any suggestion will make the subject feel relaxed, leaving you feeling wonderful. The idea of following your suggestions has become intermingled with pleasure.

And because you are controlling your awareness of those sounds, can you now make them quieter...softer... can you? ... You use your imagination to make those sounds ...far away... soft and quite... And I'm wondering does this make you relax even more... more deeply soundly relaxed...

So that you can enjoy all those positive feelings you asked for, and the more you surrender those resistances, the more room there will be inside you for pleasure, comfort and relaxation, which everyone wants,

Did the subject ask for those feelings,, I really don't remember, but the statement sounds very reasonable, so it must be Ok to feel good, to follow these suggestions to relax yes perhaps I did ask for them actually I'm going ask for them again, and again , and again,

so as you surrender to yourself you notice now that all the muscles in your head are letting go and relaxing deeply, from the forehead... those muscles above the eyebrows all the way down the face, the cheek bones...even those tiny little muscles around the mouth are letting go and relaxing deeply... letting go of tension anxiety and just relaxing deeply, you might notice a feeling of heaviness now spreading down from the face into the neck and shoulders.

Alternative wording might be *so as you surrender to my words...*

it's perfectly natural to want those feelings of pleasure... and calm and thoughtlessness to get stronger, to enjoy them more, so that the more you relax and let go the more your consciousness surrenders, and the more your subconsciousness opens itself, and you, to those pleasing feelings

The third layer has now been introduced, ***thoughtlessness***, or the idea that there is no need to think about the process. Just allow it all to happen. Later we will discuss a very powerful technique called ***The Observer Principle***, which partly incorporates the idea of thoughtlessness yet in reverse.

For the rest of this script instead of re doing the entire script I will highlight (italics) the important parts. By now you should be able to recognise the layers as they occur during the spoken script

as your body and mind **accept this comfort, allowing it to happen**...*to occur naturally, your* **subconscious can accept** *the release, from letting go, of feelings of stress and worry, fear anxiety and relax even more deeply ...soundly, and you*

Through the tops of the arms, the elbows into the wrists and the hands heavy and relaxed ...even to the very fingertips... **As you let my words into your mind, you can learn to surrender** *the stress inside you, and* **free yourself** *to enjoy relaxation, so* **if you'd like that**, *which would only be natural, then let yourself take a deep, deep breath,... and when you exhale, let your*

it with your breath, taking it away so that letting out that deep, deep breath lets you relax; **see how easy this is?**

... **In fact all you can think about is how comfortable you are and how nice it would be to just**... *drift down ... into a deep sleep... deeply soundly asleep...*

You might find your subconsciousness wanting to help your consciousness surrender, to me this has always been a very natural process *a better way of*

Deep, deep breath, and when you exhale, **let your subconscious surrender your thinking,** *so that you can be filled with deep relaxation, which is what you want anyway, isn't it?*

And you already know my words are helping you to relax and let go, don't you? Some people find the idea of hypnosis... where you are now... overwhelming, irresistible; it's as if every word I

have said, or will say gives you deeper and deeper relaxation and pleasure, and takes you further into trance, so that **you find you can easy accept any suggestions I give you as True.**

Relaxed that **nothing else matters does it**... and you want to relax and feel good **don't you**... it's a truly wonderful thing, to let go, to surrender and relax, **and this is true isn't it.**

Knowing, that every time you accept one of my suggestions, it helps you, to relax, just like you're doing now, That my suggestions help you to surrender, just like now, that my suggestions make you feel good just as you do now, **the power of all My suggestions grows,** and the pleasure grows, and your allowing yourself to let go and accept, **to take in my words my voice and suggestions becomes more complete more natural, a good thing to do.**

Almost instinctive, **existing just outside your control.** So you just **naturally choose** to **accept my suggestions** to **accept** and **invite** that comfort relaxation and pleasure **more deeply each time.**

And relax deeply now, more deeply than ever before...

The key to delivering any script with power is to understand how the mind receives information.

Our minds go through many processes when dealing with information, there is a lot around us that we are not aware of. While this subject could be a book in itself the basics are,

Can you now make them quieter...softer... can you? ... You use your imagination to make those sounds ...far away... soft and quite...

This is an example of a joined meaning sentence where you are able to say two things as one thus creating a further dual reality for the subject. The tag on the end of the statement **Can you now make them quieter...softer... can you?** Is also the first part of the next phrase **can you? ... You use your imagination to make those sounds ...far away... soft and quite...** the **can you** part carries meaning for both statements.

DELETION, DISTORTION AND GENERALIZATION

The mind will delete information that it deems unimportant or of no value to us, it will distort information in a way that helps us understand it, the mind will generalize information or match it to things we already know and understand.

Imagine that mentally you are trying to fit a square peg in a round hole, your imagination will,

One remove the peg,

Two change the shape of either the hole or the peg

Or thirdly you will convince yourself that the whole exercise is stupid and has no real value for you.

Another example you can do with your subjects, have them place a hand on the table, spreading their fingers apart, touch one finger. Now ask them which finger they are concentrating on, they will state that the finger you touched is most prominent in their mind right now. Now touch all the fingers except one. Now when you ask which finger they are focusing on it will be the one you didn't touch, the one you missed out touching. You deleted one finger and this is the one they will be now be concentrating on.

As a hypnotist this is very important information. We are going to return to this concept shortly.

DAVE ELMAN

What you are about to read is not the original Elman induction it is my version of it. There were problems with the original version. By today's standards, the Elman Induction is actually slow being fairly cumbersome. The Elman induction became popular when it was developed, way back then we didn't know as much about the human mind as we do now. If you are into history you can find the original version with much information about it online. As far as learning hypnosis goes, I recommend at least reading it.

Modern induction scripts are much faster, more reliable, many will successfully hypnotize almost anyone.

Although the Elman induction is slow by today's stage hypnotist standards it has the advantage of being easy to learn. Plus it will teach you a lot about the process and intricacies of hypnosis.

Every hypnotist should in my opinion gain some rudimentary knowledge the Elman technique as it is the basis for many of the scripts we use today. Not only that, it has the advantage of allowing you to recognize when someone is in trace, with how they behave when they are hypnotized

As you grow in experience you will eventually start creating your own inductions, each will be based on a variation of all the inductions you know, all the psychology you have incorporated with the stuff you have found to work.

For learning the basics the Elman induction is probably the best.

DAVE ELMAN INDUCTION

Once again, create a flow from the testing or convincing stage into the induction, here we will assume that the subject is sitting having just experienced the hands locked or magnetic fingers convincer...

That's excellent, now you can release your fingers and hands, the hands can relax and come apart now. I am going to show you

how to go into trance... how to relax your body and your mind... in a way that you will really enjoy....

You are setting up expectation behaviour by pre framing the subject.

Are you left or right handed, (it doesn't matter here we will assume the subject has said right handed) *ok I want you to take the right hand and make a fist for me*

Good now make that the tightest strongest fist that you can, make it so tight and so hard that not even air can get in there, really tight. Tighter and tighter so tight, so locked shut that even the atoms begin to compress and the knuckles turn white,

(Once you are satisfied that the subject is putting in a lot of effort.) *Ok just let those go, now, release it and relax the hand,*

Now you did that, I asked you to do it, but you chose to control the muscles of your hand and make it tight, you were in charge of the tension and the muscles of the hand, I might have suggested it, but you did it, you controlled through choice everything that your hand did. So, it stands to reason , that if you can make your hand tense, that you can do it in the other direction, that you can make it just as relaxed, that if you can control the tension, that you can mentally control the relaxation,

So I want you to do that for me now, as far as you went toward extreme tension go the other way and make that hand relaxed, use you mind to make that hand as relaxed as you can.

Make it so relaxed that in a moment I could pick up your hand and it would drop down again when I let go, like a rag doll, no effort and you wouldn't help me because there would be absolutely no tension in the hand at all.

(Demonstrate by lifting your own hand at the wrist, with your other hand and let it drop)

So do that for me now. Relax the whole hand from the finger tips through the palm even up to the elbow and to the shoulder.

(When you think they have got it take the wrist gently lift the hand then let go letting it drop back down.)

If they have relaxed the hand tell them "that's good" then continue, if not, (you will know because the hand won't drop back down by itself) tell them that's Ok then continue on as if everything is perfectly normal saying ...

"Isn't it amazing about humans that we can easily create tension like we did a moment ago, but when I ask you to relax... you found it more difficult, you are in control of your tension...but not your relaxation...interesting?"

Then continue

*Ok I'm going to show you something I can do, I can do this with my eyes, I can close them...make them so relaxed that they just don't want to open,,, (*show this by closing your eyes*) and I give them a little test* (raise your eyebrows as if trying to open your eyes) *but they won't open, and I stop testing them,, and I can just take it off and open my eyes again ... easy done...*

Now I want you to do that for me, just close the eyes and make them relaxed very relaxed and heavy... and when you think your there ... just give them a little test,

(Wait for them to start to move the eyebrows and immediately say

Ok stop testing, now in a moment I'm going to count to three, and when I reach three, you will take in a deep breath, open those eyes, and then as you exhale just let them close again, only this time when they close they will be twice as heavy as they are now, twice as relaxed, twice as comfortable.

Heavy and relaxed 1...2...3

As they open there eyes stare straight at the subject raise your hands and lower it as they breathe out. The idea is to get the subject to follow your hand as it lowers.

Ok now twice as heavy, deeper and more relaxed twice as relaxed as you were deeper and deeper going down now, twice as comfortable, ok that's very good you are doing really well. Now I'm going to count to three once again you will open your eyes on the count of three, and even though it may be a little harder to open them, as you breath out as you release that breath,,, just close them again, and this time you will be ten times more relaxed... ten times heavier those eyes will be heavier than ever before ten times more comfortable and deeply relaxed. Ok 1...2...3

Do the same as before raise your hand let it become the timing for them to close the eyes again,

Good deeper now ten times heavier. Ten times more relaxed

Good now I'm going to count to three again and same as before, and even though you will struggle this time open the eyes again and as you breath out just let them close down heavy and deeply relaxed, this time they will be fifty, even a hundred times more relaxed ... heavier and comfortable, in fact all you will be able to think about is how good it feels to let them go, deeply heavily relaxed so at the count of three breath in.. Open the eyes ... and as you breath out ... they become 50 times heavier, fifty times more relaxed and they shut down deeper heavier than ever before,

1..2..3.. the subject will either not open their eyes or appear to have trouble opening them either way move straight to the next part, before they are fully open.

Go deeper now deeper and sounder more and more relaxed, and as you are in control of the relaxation just make it move out ward from the eyes now, into the muscles of the face take it and control it out ward to your entire body... and once you start the process of deep relaxation, once you move it, throughout your body, no power on earth can stop you going into trance and you don't have to do anything... it will just happen... as long as you follow my instructions you will go into trance easily and quickly....

From here continue in a normal PRI fashion relaxing the whole body of the subject.

You have just learned several new skills and language patterns that can be incorporated into your hypnosis work.

THE SKILL OF FRACTIONATION

Fractionation is the process of taking the subject in then out of the state of trance in order to deepen the experience. In the case of erotic hypnosis the process can take anything from minutes, hours, even weeks. The process has been used by religious zealots to convert people to their cults or sects. During the nineties, with the wide spread use of the internet a few people began promoting seduction methods or courses based around fractionation. We being the upright noble citizens that we are will not do this.

In erotic hypnosis fractionation basically means moving the subject rapidly from a hypnotic state, to a state of being very much wide awake, then back to relaxation again. Repeating the cycle reaching deeper and deeper states.

In the Elman example these cycles move very fast, one after the other, going almost unnoticed by the subject. In the initial stages of the induction, the eyes closing several times, you are inducing a mild hypnotic state, each time you have the subject close their eyes they are going slightly deeper into trance.

Repeating an action several times trains the subject to respond. In this case repeating the eyes closed having them getting heavier three times in a sense trained the subject to relax each time they closed their eyes. There are many names for this psychological process but generally you are creating state of *Fractionation* or *Incremental Hypnosis,* where the process is broken up into easy to handle chunks, thus more easily accepted by the rational part of the mind. The more you can input a suggestion in different ways the more effective it will be.

This is going to be very important later when we discuss the art of *pre-framing* in more depth.

We have also learned how important it is to repeat suggestions. The astute student will also notice the very clever way we managed to repeat the counting down from three processes. Thus creating a trigger for later on

We have also incorporated many of the principles we discussed earlier plus a few new ones.

Inevitability Capability an advanced version of the assumption principle. Although this time it is more powerful as we have hidden a direct command within another statement

into the muscles of the face take it and control it out ward to your entire body... and once you start the process of deep relaxation, once you move it, throughout your body, no power on earth can stop you going into trance and you don't have to do anything... it will just happen... as long as you follow my instructions you will go into trance easily and quickly....

Realistically this is a pretty big assumption, that no power on earth will stop you, yet at the same time it's going to be easy. In fact we are creating a sense of the inevitable within the subject *as long as you follow my instructions you will go into trance easily and quickly.*

The remainder of the inductions in this section are basically standard fair, I believe that you now have enough information with enough insight, to expand on them yourself adjusting them to your style. I repeat again, practise, practise, practise use each of them at least once to get a feel for it, I often find that after years of avoiding particular inductions, simply because I didn't like it, once I've adapted it, made it my own or combined parts of it with other inductions, they are all effective in some way.

NONVERBAL SHIFTS

Before we move to these inductions however let's learn some more stuff.

The next two inductions involve the use of the ***Unconscious Behaviour*** of your subject.

In NLP there is a lot of talk about building rapport, (I'm almost positive I will write a book on this one day) Part of attaining good rapport with your subject is the *pacing* or *mirroring* of the subject's behaviour. Standard NLP or sales courses will talk about this in great detail. Matching the body language or speech patterns of your prospect. However in the field of hypnosis, especially erotic hypnosis we are going to do this outside of our subjects own conscious awareness.

For example by a subtly almost imperceivable matching the subject's breathing pattern, facial expressions, body or face touches, you will have mirrored a part of them that is not in their conscious awareness. The trick here is to be aware of what is within their awareness. Mirroring a persons seated position or the way they cross their legs is something they are most likely aware or conscious of.

While their breathing or how often we scratch our face during the day, is outside our normal awareness. Scratching, eye contact, arm or leg crossing, foot or hand movement's slips past our awareness. These little subtle actions or habits goes mostly unnoticed. It is these unnoticed behaviours that you as a hypnotist will notice then begin to subtly mirror.

Mirroring and pacing, is effective only to the degree that it remains out of the subject's consciousness. However *Nonverbal Shifts* are indicative of many subjective qualities, when properly understood.

NONVERBAL INDUCTION

The subject is seated in a chair and instructed to hold both arms out in front of them and upward so that the hands are slightly above eye level. They should be parallel, the hands being shoulder width apart. The hypnotist now moves back and forth in front of the subject from one side to the other, making a small postural change in the subject's right arm first, then over to the other side to make a similar charge in the left arm.

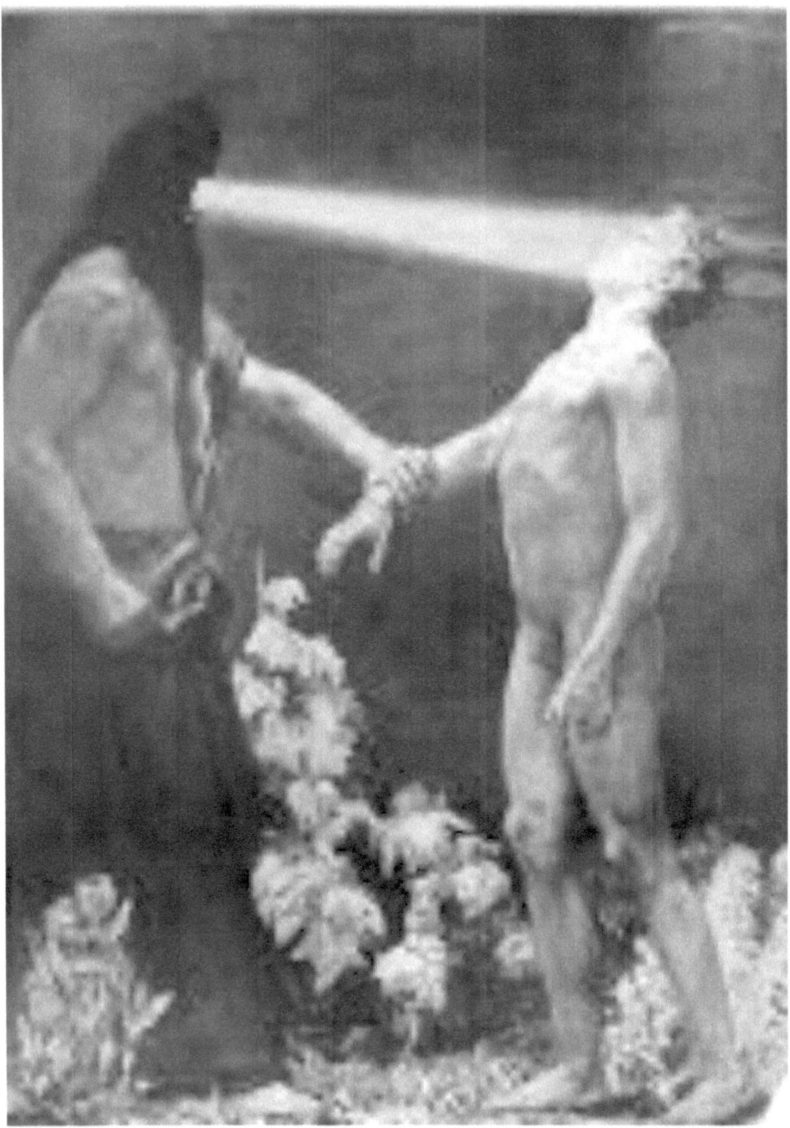

First the right arm is bent at the elbow so that the hand comes a bit inward and downward (the right elbow simultaneously extending more outward). The hypnotist then moves over to the left side and repeats the movement of the subject's left arm in the same way. After each movement he pauses a few seconds and observes the posture.

This permits him both to observe the subject's reaction and to allow time for adjustment to the new change in posture.

Once again he moves to the subject's right side and adjusts the right arm again slightly downward. This is then matched in a few seconds with a similar adjustment in the left hand. The postural adjustments of the arms and hands are constantly transmitting the message of "inward and downward," inward into one's self, and downward toward a more unconscious level of awareness.

Finally, when the hands are almost together and are barely above the lap the hypnotist grasps both of them firmly by the wrist and forcibly lowers them rapidly all the way down. At this point the subject's eyes will usually close and his head slump forward on his chest. If this does not happen the hypnotist can pull the eyelids down, and by a push on the back of the head, administer this final forceful suggestion which implies, "Go inward and downward, close your eyes and enter a deep relaxed, hypnotic state!"

No words have been spoken, but the induction has been accomplished by the series of progressively spaced changes in posture. To remove the hypnotic state which has been so achieved the hypnotist simply reverses the movements. First, he lifts up the head. Then he lifts up both arms to the position they held just prior to the forcible lowering of them. Next, one arm and hand at a time the movements are reversed. The movements are now outward and upward, "Come up out of yourself and back into the conscious state," is the message. Finally, the arms are back in their original position; the patient's eyes are fully open, the head is up.

ANOTHER NON-VERBAL INDUCTION

This is another classic it has been used by hypnotists all over the world for more years than I can count, it is particularly effective when language is a barrier, rather than calling in an interpreter try this method

Start as follows" *I would like you to simply allow things to take place. Do not try to make anything happen, but do not try to stop things from taking place. Is this agreeable to you?*

Take the subject's hand as if you were going to be shaking hands. Have the subject's arm stretched straight out.

With the subject looking directly in your eyes, begin slowly raising, and lowering the arm about three to four inches each way. Keep your eyes fixed on the client's eyes.

As the subject begins to blink their eyes, interrupt your up, and down movement of the arm, and begin pushing the arm down slightly.

Return to the up, and down movements of the arm until the client blinks again. Once again, when the subject blinks their eyes push the arm down slightly.

You will discover that within a few movements the eyes will close completely. Drop their arm to their side.

THE GIL BOYNE INDUCTION

The Gil Boyne induction is another good one to practise with, it combines many elements from other inductions. Primarily it is a *progressive relation induction* with various *language patterns* plus some *kinetic techniques.* As it is a classic I am presenting it here in its original form. Later I will revisit this induction as it is particularly good for adapting to erotic work

You are about to enjoy a very pleasant and a very beneficial experience. Subject is seated

Now stretch out on your back, with your legs separated, so that no parts of your calves or thighs are touching. Keep feet separated at least 8 to 10 inches; arms extended loosely and limply alongside your body, palms facing downward and fingers limply outstretched.

Once we begin, you can help by remaining quiet and passive. Our first goal is for you to become unaware of your body. You can best achieve that goal by avoiding movement.

The first thing that I want you to do is to fix your eyes at a spot on the ceiling overhead. Pick out an imaginary spot, and stare at that spot without moving a muscle.

Now, take a deep breath and fill up your lungs. Exhale slowly. Sleep now.

Now, take a second and even deeper breath. Take in all the air that your lungs can hold. Exhale slowly. Sleep now.

Now, let your eyelids close down. Now, your eyelids are closed down. Please leave them closed down until I ask you to open them again. You will always be able to open your eyes, unless I was to give you a direct command and tell you that your eyelids are locked closed. And I don't intend to do that. Hypnosis is a state of mind, not a state of eyelids.

Now, I want you to mentally picture and imagine that you are looking at the muscles in the tips of the toes of your left foot. In your imagination, follow those muscles as they move back into the ball of the foot. In your imagination, follow those muscles as they move back into the ball of the foot. Back into the arch, and all the way back into the heel. Now, turn all those muscles loose. Let them grow limp and lazy, just like a handful of loose rubber bands.

Now, as the muscles begin to relax, just let your mind relax, too. Let your mind drift where it will. Let your mind drift off to pleasant scenes in your imagination.

And now, let the relaxation move on up, into the ankle now. From the ankle, all the way up to the left knee. The calf muscles begin to grow loose and limp—heavy, and so relaxed.

All of your tensions are fading away. You're relaxing more with each easy breath that you take. Begin breathing more deeply, now, just as you breathe each night, when you are deep and sound in slumber. Just imagine that you can see your breath as a white mist, coming from your nostrils. Each and every time that you exhale this white mist, you are freeing yourself of tension, and going deeper, deeper into drowsy relaxation.

Now, from the knee, all the way to the left hip, the long thigh muscles are turning loose, easing off, and just relaxing now. Now, as those muscles relax, just let go a little more, and gently, calmly, easily, drift on over, into a pleasant state of easy relaxation.

Now let the wave of relaxation that started from the toes of your left foot just a few seconds ago—let it move over now into the toes of the right foot, back into the arch, and all the way back to the heel. Turn all of those muscles loose, and go deeper and deeper into relaxation.

Into the ankle, the muscles let go. From the ankle, all the way up to the right knee. The calf muscles are turning loose and letting go.

You're relaxing more with each easy breath that you take. With each sound that you hear. Each sound carries you deeper, deeper and sounder in sleep.

From the knee, all the way up to the right hip. The long thigh muscles grow limp and lazy. Now, as those muscles relax, just go all the way down, deeper and deeper in drowsy slumber.

Turn them all loose and go deeper in sleep.

Now, the wave of relaxation moves on up, into the stomach now. Into the solar plexus, the centre of nervous energy. Each muscle and nerve lets loose the tensions, relaxing. You're drifting down, deeper and deeper in sleep. Down, deeper in slumber.

Up through the ribs, the muscles relax. Into the broad muscles of the chest. The muscles of the chest grow limp and loose, and so relaxed. All of your tensions are fading away.

You're relaxing now, more with each easy beat of your heart, and going deeper in drowsy slumber.

Into the neck, the muscles let go. All around the neck, the muscles relax, just as they relax each night when you are deep and sound in sleep. Turn them all loose, and go deeper and deeper in slumber. Now let the relaxation start down your back. From the base of the skull to the base of the spine. Each muscle and nerve along the spine lets loose the tension, relaxing. You're drifting down. Deeper and deeper in sleep. Down deeper in drowsy slumber.

And the wave of relaxation spreads out into the broad muscles of the back. All across the small of the back. All across the back of the shoulders. Turn loose every muscle and every nerve in the back, and go deeper and deeper in sleep.

Into the shoulder, the muscles let go. From the shoulders, down to the elbows of both arms. The upper arm muscles are turning loose, easing off, and just relaxing now.

From the elbows, down to the wrists on both arms, the forearm muscles grow limp and lazy.

From the wrists to the fingertips of hands, each muscle and nerve lets loose the tensions, relaxing, you're drifting down. Deeper and deeper in sleep.

Into the jaws, the muscles relax. The jaws are parting slightly, teeth not quite touching. All around the mouth, the muscles let go.

Up through the nose, each nerve gives way. All around the eyes, the muscles are heavy, and so relaxed. Even your eyebrows are relaxing now. Across the forehead, the muscles smooth out. Across the top of the skull. Down the back of the neck. Down through the temples, back around the ears, all of the muscles are loose, and lazy—just like a handful of loose rubber bands.

And you may feel now, a pleasant tingling sensation in the tips of your toes, or in your fingertips—a pleasant tingling sensation, growing stronger and stronger now, as your entire body is being bathed in the pleasant glow of complete and utter relaxation.

Now you are completely relaxed. Each muscle and nerve in your body is loose and limp and relaxed, and you feel good.

TWO-FINGER TECHNIQUE

Subject is seated

For the moment, rest your arms limply on your thighs, just like this (demonstrate position to subject). *Now I want you to look out here at my hand. In a moment I'm going to bring my hand up in front of your eyes like this. (Demonstrate bringing index and middle finger of right hand, in a pointing V position, to a position just above their eyebrows) When I do, I'll pass my hand down in front of your eye. Keep your eyes fixed on my fingers. As I pass my hand down, let your eyelids close down. (Bring hand straight down, one finger moving down over each eye)*

(Move fingers to a pointing V position just above eyebrows so they have to look up at an angle to see fingertips) All right, now fix your eyes on my fingers. Now I'm passing my hand down in front of your eyes, and as I do, let your eyelids close down. (Move hand straight down, one finger moving down over each eye)

Now your eyelids are closed down. I want you to relax every tiny muscle and nerve in and around your eyelids. I want you to relax them so much that they wouldn't work even if you wanted them to.

Now, when you know that you've relaxed them that much that they wouldn't work even if you wanted them to, test them; you'll see you've been completely successful. Now, relax them so much that they wouldn't work even if you wanted them to. Now test them; you'll see you've been completely successful. (If they open their eyes, tell them to relax them again, this time more completely and test again. If they don't open their eyes, pause three seconds and continue)

All right, that's fine. Now, stop trying and just relax and go deeper now. Now I'm going to raise your hand. I will do it by grasping your right thumb in my fingers like this. (Grasp thumb between thumb and index finger—make sure you grasp the correct thumb) As I lift your hand, just let it hang limply in my fingers

(Optional: slightly rock arm back and forth) Then, when I drop it, let it drop like a wet, limp rag. When you hand touches your body, as it drops, send a wave or relaxation from the top of your head all the way down to the tips of your toes. This will double your present level of relaxation.

(Lift hand, optionally rocking it) *Now, I'm raising your hand. That's it, let it hang limply. That's good. Now, when I drop it, let it drop like a limp, wet rag, and as it touches your body, send a wave of relaxation from the top of your head to the tip of your toes.* (Drop hand) *That's good.*

Now, we'll do that again with the left hand. Now I'm going to pick up your left hand, and as I take your thumb, just let it hang limply. (Optional: slightly rock arm back and forth) That's good; now you're getting the idea. When I drop it, let it drop like a wet, limp rag. When it touches your body, send another wave or relaxation from the top of your head to the tips of your toes and double your present level of relaxation. (Drop hand) That's good.

Now, your body is relaxed and I'm going to show you how to relax your mind. Listen very carefully. The next time I touch your forehead, I want you to begin counting from one hundred backward in this way: One hundred, deeper asleep. Ninety-nine, deeper asleep. Ninety-eight, deeper asleep, and so on. After counting just a few numbers, by the time you reach ninety-seven, or ninety-six, or maybe, at the most, ninety-five, you will find those numbers disappearing. You will find your mind has become so relaxed that you'll just relax them out of your mind.

All right, get ready now, three, two, and one. (Tap subject on forehead) *Begin counting. (Listen to them count down. Based upon the rate of speed, you may say the following statement) Good, slow them down now.* (After each count, say one of the following) *good/ fine.* (After the count of ninety-seven say) *Start relaxing them out of your mind. (After several more counts, based on how the subject is performing, say) Let them relax out of your mind right now. (After another count) Let them fade away completely.*

(After subject has stopped counting, continue with) *That's fine, you've relaxed your body; you've relaxed your mind; you've gone into a much deeper state of hypnosis.*

By now you will have noticed a lot of reoccurring themes and ideas in each of the inductions, those principles should remain consistent in all good inductions. Even when examining newer inductions these tried and true techniques are still found. So we will now look at a few different ways of doing inductions.

CONFUSION INDUCTION

There are many ideas about what exactly constitutes the hypnotic state, some say it is a focused attention, other schools of thought explain it as a state of confusion, a state where the mind doesn't know what to do next so it shuts down or drifts off, to avoid any further confusion.

The basic message to this induction is the **conscious forgetting**, while the *subconscious remembers*.

We are effectively taking the conscious mind in one direction, while the subconscious mind is directed in another direction. There is some argument as to what this confusion technique really is.

Are we capturing the subconscious minds attention, making it focus on something while dismissing the conscious attention, is this really confusion or are we creating a state of mental fatigue.

All arguments aside the following is a powerful induction it is well worth the time to study

For this induction you will want to adjust your speech, speak slowly, rhythmically. Have the subject sit or lay in a relaxed position, with their eyes closed.

Just close those eyelids and let your mind drift where it will.

You are aware of everything, and yet you are not aware. You are listening with your subconscious mind, while your conscious mind

is far away, and not listening. Your conscious mind is far away, and not listening. Your subconscious mind is awake, and listening, and hearing everything while your conscious mind remains very relaxed and peaceful. You can relax peacefully because your subconscious mind is taking charge, and when this happens, you close your eyes and let your subconscious do all the listening. Your subconscious mind knows, and because you're subconscious mind knows, your conscious mind does not need to know and can stay asleep, and not mind while your subconscious mind stays wide awake.

You have much potential in your subconscious mind which you don't have in your conscious mind. You can remember everything that has happened with your subconscious mind, but you cannot remember everything with your conscious mind. You can forget so easily, and with forgetting certain things you can remember other things. Remembering what you need to remember, and forgetting what you can forget. It does not matter if you forget, you need not remember. Your subconscious mind remembers everything that you need to know and you can let your subconscious mind listen and remember while your conscious mind sleeps and forgets. Keep your eyes closed, and listen with your subconscious mind, and when you're listening very, very carefully, your head can nod "yes".

As you continue to listen to me, with your subconscious mind, your conscious mind sleeps deeper and deeper, and deeper, and deeper. Let your conscious mind stay deeply asleep, and let your subconscious mind listen to me.

You have much potential in your subconscious mind which you don't have in your conscious mind. You can remember everything that has happened with your subconscious mind, but you cannot remember everything with your conscious mind. You can forget so easily, and with forgetting certain things you can remember other things. Remembering what you need to remember, and forgetting what you can forget. It does not matter if you forget, you need not remember. Your subconscious mind remembers everything that you need to know and you can let your subconscious mind listen and remember while your conscious mind sleeps and forgets. Keep your eyes closed, and listen with your subconscious mind, and when you're listening very, very carefully, your head can now "yes".

As you continue to listen to me, with your subconscious mind, your conscious mind sleeps deeper and deeper, and deeper, and deeper. Let your conscious mind stay deeply asleep, and let your subconscious mind listen to me.

If you were a little confused reading this...good, imagine how confused your subject will be, in that confusing they won't be thinking about much at all, thus leaving the mind open to suggestion.

ASSOCIATION INDUCTION

In this induction you are forcing the subject to associate various feelings or natural responses to hypnosis or the trance state. A sample of this technique is the association we make with darkened rooms, laying down, closing our eyes and getting ready for sleep. All these are things we do that signal the brain it is time to sleep.

You can close your eyes now ... And begin breathing deeply and slowly ... Before you let go completely, and go into a deep hypnotic state, just let yourself listen carefully to everything I say to you ...

It's going to happen automatically ... So you don't need to think about that now ... And you will have no conscious control over what happens...

The muscles in and around your eyes will relax all by themselves as you continue breathing ... Easily and freely...

Without thinking about it, you will soon enter a deep, peaceful, hypnotic trance, without any effort ... There is nothing important for your conscious mind to do...

There is nothing really important except the activities of your subconscious mind ... And that can be just as automatic as dreaming ... And you know how easily you can forget your dreams when you awaken...

You are responding very well. Without noticing it, you have already altered your rate of breathing ... You are breathing much more easily and freely ... And you are revealing signs that indicate you are beginning to drift into a hypnotic trance...

You can really enjoy relaxing more and more, and your subconscious mind will listen to each word I say ... And it keeps becoming less important for you to consciously listen to my voice...

Your subconscious mind can hear even if I whisper...

You are continuing to drift into a more detached state as you examine privately in your own mind ... Secrets, feelings, sensations, and behaviour you didn't know you had ... At the same time, letting go completely ... Your own mind is solving that problem ... At your own pace ... Just as rapidly as it feels you are ready ...

You continue becoming more relaxed and comfortable as you sit there with your eyes closed...

As you experience that deepening comfort you don't have to move, or talk, or let anything bother you...

Your own inner mind can respond automatically to everything I tell you ... and you will be pleasantly surprised with your continuous progress... You are getting much closer to a deep hypnotic trance ... And you are beginning to realize that you don't care whether or not you are going into a deep trance...

Being in this peaceful state enables you to experience the comfort of the hypnotic trance...

Being hypnotized is always a very enjoyable, very pleasant, calm, peaceful, completely relaxing experience...

It seems natural ... to include hypnosis in your future...

Every time I hypnotize you it keeps becoming more enjoyable, and you continue experiencing more benefits ... So you will really enjoy having me hypnotize you...

You will always enjoy the sensations ... Of comfort ... Of peacefulness ... Of calmness ... And all the other sensations that come automatically from this wonderful experience...

You will be really happy that you decided to have me hypnotize you ...as you continue experiencing progressive understanding on your part...

You are learning something about yourself ... You are developing your own techniques of therapy ... Without knowing you are developing them ...You can have it as a surprise sooner or later ... a very pleasant surprise ...

Imagine yourself in a place you like very much ... By a lake, or by the ocean ... Perhaps you are floating gently on a sailboat on a peaceful lake ... On a warm, summer day ... You are continuing to relax even more now ... And you continue becoming more comfortable ...

This is your own world that you like very much...

You are going to find that any time you want to spend a few minutes by yourself, relaxing, and feeling very comfortable and serene, you can automatically go back to this feeling you're experiencing now...

You can put yourself into this world anytime you like ... There are times when you will want this serene feeling ... And it is yours whenever you want it ...

Continue enjoying this pleasant experience as your subconscious mind is receiving everything I tell you ... And you will be pleased the way you automatically respond to everything I say.

If you read the association induction carefully you will be able to see how this (and a few others can be easily adapted to erotic work, it will be not hard at all to convert or adjust those subtle phrasings to have the client enter an aroused hypnotic state. Here are a few examples, of how the subject can be taken toward association.

Before you let go completely, and go into a deep hypnotic state, just let yourself listen carefully to everything I say to you...

This instructs the subject as explained earlier, the command phase is to listen carefully. Using the word *carefully* implies that something might be important. We are trained even as children that things we need to be careful with are important things.

It's going to happen ***automatically...***

So you don't need to think about that now...

This is entrainment one used by religion for centuries, plus it provides you with an out, *don't think about it, if you really want you can think about it later.*

You are responding very well. Without noticing it, you have already altered your rate of breathing ... You are breathing much more easily and freely ... And you are revealing signs that indicate you are beginning to drift into a hypnotic trance...

Here you are obviously watching the subject, taking note of any reactions, slumping of the shoulders eyes flickering shifting position whatever it is you are making the subject believe that these signs mean hypnosis.

You can really enjoy relaxing more and more, and your subconscious mind will listen to each word I say ... And it keeps becoming less important for you to consciously listen to my voice...

Your subconscious mind can hear even if I whisper... recognise the double bind?

You are continuing to drift into a more detached state as you examine privately in your own mind ... Secrets, feelings, sensations, and behaviour you didn't know you had ... At the same time, letting go completely ... Your own mind is solving that problem ... At your own pace ... Just as rapidly as it feels you are ready ...

This could easily be adapted to an erotic situation, in fact if you are in this situation assuming you have pre-framed correctly your subject will think this is perhaps what you are referring to. The idea of ***Secrets, feelings, sensations, and behaviour*** can be very powerful if the subject already has disposed themselves to the idea that this is an erotic session.

You get the idea, there are a lot more principles in this script. As in the others some more are examined in the following inductions.

ARM DROP INDUCTION

Your subject is asked to raise an arm so that the hand is slightly above the head and given suggestions. There are a number of aspects of this induction which we have examined before that can be used to make this a very powerful and effective induction.

First, the subjects arm is sneakily placed in such a position that eventually enough physical fatigue will set in that they won't be able to hold it up anyway.

This natural fatigue is matched to suggestions such as ***going "down" into a heavier and heavier, "deep state of relaxation."*** The harder the individual keeps fighting to hold their arm up, the more difficult it becomes. The act of fighting against fatigue and strain actually causes more fatigue and strain.

We spoke before of ***implied information*** how something that is implied or indirectly stated can often be more powerful than a direct statement or command. The more your subject is consciously committed to the proposition implied by the statement that, ***"You will not go into a deep state of relaxation until the arm is all the way down."*** This **implies**, by default that, ***"You will go into such a state when the arm comes all the way down."***

Have subject raise arm so that hand is slightly above head, begin as follows

Stare at one of your fingers, either the index or the middle finger. You may continue to look at it, or, if you wish, close your eyes and visualize it in your mind's eye.

As you fixate your gaze on it you will notice that the other fingers tend to fade out of focus and that your entire arm begins to feel heavier and heavier. The longer you concentrate on that finger the heavier and heavier your arm becomes.

But you will not go into a deep state of relaxation until the arm has come all the way down. Keep concentrating on that finger while the arm gets heavier and heavier and heavier. (When downward movement become apparent) *Notice that as the arm is getting heavier it is slowly coming down, down, down. But you will not go into a deep and profound state of relaxation until the arm is all the way down. Going... down... down, down... deeper... deeper... and deeper.* Continue with deepening suggestions: The suggestions must be timed with the actual movement of the subjects arm, also if possible to the out breath.

ARM LEVITATION INDUCTION

Let's continue in this same vain creating a link between what is happening to the subject, their feelings, their thoughts, while tying these into the actual process of hypnosis. This induction can also be used as a deepening technique. It requires that you pay special attention to your subject's reactions and responses, pacing your suggestions to the responses of your subject.

Subject is sitting comfortable arms resting on the armrests of a chair

I'm going to count from one up to twenty. As I do, a light, easy, pleasant feeling moves into your right hand and into your right arm. As I continue counting, that feeling grows stronger and stronger. Soon you'll feel the first slight movement of your fingers, a twitching of the muscles. (At this point, grasp the subjects arm and demonstrate how it will move as you continue with the following suggestions by slowing raising it upward). *Then your hand begins to lift. Your arm begins to lift. It continues moving, lifting, and rising until it comes to rest upon your chest.*

Now when you feel the movement in your hand and in your arm, don't try to resist. You could resist if you chose to, that is not why you are here. Just let your subconscious mind do its perfect work. All right, now we are ready to begin.

Number One - The first light, easy sensation moves into the fingertips of your right hand.

Number Two - The feeling is spreading around beneath the fingernails.

Number Three - It is moving up to the first joint of the fingers.

Number Four - Spreading to the large knuckle across the back of the hand.

Number Five - the first slight movements begin to start taking place. Slight movements of the fingers, a twitching of the muscles.

Number Six - The light sensation spreads all across the back of your hand.

Number Seven - Spreading over and into your thumb.

Number Eight - Moving now all through the palm of your hand.

Number Nine - The light sensation spreads up and into your wrist. Think of your left hand now. You'll see by comparison, your left hand is beginning to feel very, very heavy.

While on Number Ten your right hand grows lighter and lighter with each number I count; just as light as a feather floating in the breeze and even lighter. As light as a gas-filled balloon. Just as a gas-filled balloon will rise and float towards the ceiling, in the same way, by the time I reach the count of twenty, your right hand is moving, lifting, rising and floating.

Number Eleven - The light sensation has moved beyond your wrist now, spreading into your forearm.

Twelve, Thirteen - Once again, think of your left hand. Your left hand has grown so heavy, it feels as though it were made of marble or stone.

Fourteen - That light sensation is spreading up toward your elbow.

Now on Fifteen - From the fingertips all the way up to the elbow your hand has grown light, light and free. It's beginning to lift. It's moving, lifting, rising and floating.

(At this point, if the hand is not moving, gently lift the hand to get it started)

All right, sixteen - Now your arm is moving and lifting and rising. And as your arm is lifting, you're going deeper and deeper into hypnosis.

Seventeen - Your hand continues moving, lifting and rising now until it comes to rest over on your body.

Eighteen - Moving, lifting, rising, and floating. Right on over now and when your hand comes to rest upon your body, at that time your eyelids lock tightly closed. Your eyelids lock so tightly closed at that point, the more you try to open them the tighter they're locking closed.

Nineteen - Your hand is getting ready to come down and rest upon your body.

Twenty - Now your hand has come to rest upon your body and at the same time, your eyelids are locked so tightly closed, the more you try to open your eyelids the tighter they are locking closed.

That's fine, stop trying and go deeper into trance.

MOUNTAIN TRIP INDUCTION

Depending on your subject's needs or your personal taste you may want to experiment with more descriptive inductions. Don't get too wrapped up in the words, use your own language and descriptions. Once again this induction assumes that you have done a test or two on your subject, they are ready to be hypnotised.

Continue inhaling deeply and exhaling slowly about five or six times ... each time you exhale your whole body keeps relaxing more, you continue feeling more calm, more peaceful and more at ease ...

As you continue relaxing, I want you to use your imagination. Imagine yourself lying on the grass in a soft, green meadow, the sun is shining gently, and there is an easy breeze blowing over your body ... you continue feeling more comfortable and at ease ...

Beautiful flowers are blooming all around you ... you can see the flowers moving gently in the breeze ... notice the wonderful fragrance of the flowers ...

Now, in your mind I want you to stand up ... look to the north and see the beautiful mountain at the end of this meadow ... let's take a trip up that mountain ... you look around and notice an easy flowing stream to the right of you ... you are walking over to the stream, and you bend over and put your hand in the water. You notice the water is pure, clean, cool and refreshing. Listen to the gentle flow of the rapids...

Since the stream seems to come from the mountains, let's follow the stream up into the mountains ... as we move along, following the stream, we come to a pond at the head of the stream ... you bend over and put your hand into the water and you notice it is nice and warm ... since at this level of your mind you are an excellent swimmer, we decide to get in the water and swim for a brief time ... you can feel the warm water surrounding your body as you quietly move through the water ... it feels so refreshing and so enjoyable, but it's time to get out now and continue moving up the mountain ... as we climb, you can hear the birds chirping ... you smell the pine trees ... once in a while you can still see the meadow in small openings between the trees ... we're halfway up the mountain now ... we notice a fallen tree over on the left and we decide to stop and rest ... the meadow below is in full view from here ... the scene is really beautiful ... now it's time to continue on up the mountain ...

you can imagine how beautiful it will be to be at the top to be able to look down into the meadow below ...

The breeze is blowing gently, and you can notice the smell of small cedar trees as we are nearing the top of the mountain ... just a few more steps and we will be at the top ... we finally made it ... you can see the deep canyon on the other side ... and from this side you can see the meadow below ...

Just ahead, you notice a sign there on top of the mountain ... you walk over to it and you notice that it says, "Speak the questions you want answered most into the canyon below, and you will see the answer written in the sky above" ...

You are deciding the most important question that you want to speak into the canyon below ... as soon as you make that decision, you ask the question and then look to the sky above for your answer ... (Pause for a minute or two for subject to receive answer)

Now it's time to go back down the mountain and return to the meadow ... you can notice the sun beginning to set on the hills on the left ... we still have plenty of time to get down before it gets dark, but we need to be on our way down ...

As we're going down, we notice a few deer off in the forest ... we're halfway down now ... we pause for a few minutes and sit on the fallen tree again ... we can see the beautiful sunset as it is forming ... now we continue moving on down ... you can hear the birds chirping ... now we come to the pond, and we can see the reflection of the sunset on the surface of the water ... we continue on, following the beautiful, refreshing stream ... now we're back in the meadow, and you lie down in the comfortable grass again ... you can smell the fragrance of the flowers ... and now you are ready to receive some additional suggestions I will be giving you before you awaken from the hypnotic state.

MISDIRECTION OF THE IMAGINATION INDUCTION

There will be occasions when your subject, is just not into it, in normal life this means no go, in the M\s D\s relationship however the rules are somewhat different. If you need this explained to you, then you might be reading the wrong book.

If your subject is not in the mood this induction is good as it misdirects the purpose of the exercise, it *"appears"* to be a test of the imagination

Have subject sit relaxed, hands on knees, body relaxed and passive

Just sit and relax Do you have a good imagination? (If subject responds "Yes", continue, if the subject responds "No", simply state that they are too hard on themselves and continue) ***In other words, can you close your eyes and imagine a scene, visualize a scene and see it in front of your eyes?*** (Once again, continue on "Yes", deal with "No") ***Good. Let's test your imagination in a few ways. I'll describe what I want you to visualize and then after you close your eyes and you visualize it, I'll ask you a few questions about what you see.***

(The following is a sample scene and questions. If the subject doesn't "drive" adapt some other activity that the subject is familiar with)

Do you drive a car? (If "Yes", continue, else find another topic) ***Alright, close your eyelids down and imagine you're standing in front of your car. Now when you see it very clearly, just nod your head*** (Wait for nod) ***Fine, now you're looking at your car, what colour is it? (Wait for response) Good. Open the door of the car and get in behind the wheel. Now look straight ahead. Is the speedometer in the centre or to your right or to your left?*** (Wait for response) ***Is the speedometer circular, semi-circular, horizontal or vertical?*** (Wait for response) ***Alright, what colour is the needle that indicates the speed on the speedometer?*** (Wait for response)

Alright, fine. Open your eyes. Could you see all that clearly? (Wait for response) ***Now let's test your imagination in another way.***

We learned a couple of things about your imagination right then. This time when you close your eyelids right down, imagine you're at a swimming place, a beach, a pool, a lake or at the ocean. Close your eyelids down.

Now I want you to imagine that you're at a swimming place. When you see the scene clearly in your mind's eye, nod your head (Wait for head to nod) *Alright, fine. Now look around you at this place and tell me what you see* (Wait for description) *Do you see any people there?* (If "Yes", say the following *"Pick out one of the persons and describe them to me"*, if "No", have subject describe some item that he saw at scene)

(This section is the actual misdirection) *That's very good, open your eyes. Could you see all that clearly as a mental picture? That showed that you have a good imagination to create, because in that instance I asked you something where you had to create the scenes in the picture. Now we'll go to the other extreme and find out how well you can imagine a simple, single object. This time when you close your eyelids down, imagine that you're looking at a full moon.*

Close your eyelids down. Now then I want you to imagine that you are either seated outside or in a car, or at the beach, or maybe looking out your bedroom window. Its night time and you're looking up at a full moon. To help you to see the full moon, I want you to now to roll your eyeballs back up, with your eyelids remaining closed down. Roll your eyeballs backup in your head as if you could see the full moon right up here (Touch subjects forehead lightly) backup in the centre of your forehead.

(Pick up the pace slightly and read this section as one flowing sentence) *Roll your eyeballs way back up in your head and as you do your eyelids lock tightly closed the more you try to open them the tighter they are locking closed try now to open your eyelids they're locking tighter and tighter, now stop trying, just relax and sleep. Let a good and pleasant feeling now come all over your body. Let every muscle and nerve in your body go limp and loose. Breathe easily and deeply and send a way of deep relaxation from the top of your head to the top of your toes.*

FOREST AND STREAM INDUCTION

For this classic induction it is helpful to have background ambient music sounds of, birds, or other forest sound effects, playing ever so softly. However do not start the music until indicated.

Proceed as follows

Get yourself in just as comfortable a position as you can...

Now close your eyes and inhale deeply and hold it for three or four seconds and then exhale slowly ... (Pause as subject does this and just in case you have forgotten those **three dots** mean that you should be timing the next phrase to your subjects outward breath)

Again breathe in deeply and exhale slowly ... keep doing that 5 or 6 more times...

As you inhale, you bring more oxygen into your body, and as you exhale it causes your body to keep relaxing more and more ... (Pause and observe)

Now you can continue breathing easily and freely, and can feel yourself becoming more calm and peaceful...

You are revealing signs that indicate you are moving into a very deep, peaceful state of relaxation ... as I continue talking to you, you can keep relaxing more peacefully ... not caring how deeply you relax, just happy to continue becoming more calm, more peaceful, and more at ease ... continuing to breathe easily and freely ...

Your subconscious mind will always be aware of what I'm saying to you, so it keeps becoming less and less important for you to consciously listen to my voice...

Your subconscious mind, and all levels of your inner mind can hear and receive everything I tell you, and your conscious mind can relax completely...

You are continuing to experience perfect peace of mind, and can feel yourself moving into the situation I describe to you ... it's going to happen automatically, and you don't even need to think about it consciously...

(Start background tape. Pause your speaking for about 30 seconds after starting background sounds)

Now I want you to imagine yourself lying in a comfortable position near a stream of fresh, clear water, in a beautiful forest on a perfect summer day...

There is a warm, gentle breeze, and the air is fresh and clean, the sound of the peaceful stream is very relaxing...

It keeps becoming less important for you to consciously listen to my voice because your subconscious mind and all levels of your inner mind are hearing and receiving everything I say...

In your mind, you are enjoying the beauty of nature, as the sunlight shines through the trees and you listen to the gentle flow of water and the birds singing cheerfully...

You are lying there; comfortably relaxing ... it is so peaceful that you continue feeling more relaxed than ever before in your entire life...

As you continue enjoying this peaceful, pleasant experience, a soothing drowsiness is coming over your whole body, from the top of your head to the bottom of your feet...

You continue feeling calmer, more relaxed and more secure...

And now, as you lie there with your eyes closed, you are so relaxed and comfortable and happy that you continue moving into a more peaceful, more detached state...

It may seem like you are drifting into a state of sleep...

There may be times when it seems like my voice is a long distance away ... and there may be times, when I'm talking to you, that you will not be consciously aware of my voice, and that's okay, because your subconscious mind is still receiving every word I say, and is making true everything I tell you ...

From now on you will be influenced only by positive thoughts, ideas and feelings...

The following thoughts come to you ... I am calm, secure, and relaxed ... I am comfortable and at ease ... I am in control of myself at all times ... I am responsible for my body, and will always treat my body well ... my mind enables me to be relaxed and calm as I go about the activities of my daily life ...

Your subconscious mind and all levels of your inner mind can now review and examine what has caused that problem, and can assess that information and work out a solution that is pleasing to you...

And you will be pleased to notice yourself improving more each day, and you can be sure it is permanent and lasting ...

When your inner mind understands what has caused that problem and realizes that it is okay for you to get rid of that problem, one of the fingers on your right hand will lift up towards the ceiling and will remain up until I tell it to go back down.

OBJECT DROP INDUCTION

This is one of my favourite inductions simply because it is fun, it has a physical element to it that signals the subject to go into trance. It can be done with just about anything from a pen, a pencil or a coin.

Ask the subject to get a pen, pencil or coin to hold it out in front of the body between the thumb and index finger. Tell them to grip it in a secure way.

Now close your eyes and think of that (pen or pencil, coin) between the thumb and index finger of your right hand ... Now breathe in deeply and exhale slowly five times ... Each time you inhale you bring more oxygen into your lungs. It passes from your lungs into your heart, and your heart pumps it into your circulatory system. It moves through your whole body, and each time you exhale you keep relaxing, becoming calmer and more peaceful.

You might even for a moment forget that you were holding the pen...

But now you remember...

That relaxation is moving through your whole body, and through your right shoulder, down your arm into your hand and fingers ... soon the fingers on your right hand will become so relaxed that the (pen or pencil, coin) will slip from your hand and drop to the floor.

As you hear the (pens or pencils, coins) dropping to the floor, it may seem a little humorous at first, but it will cause you to continue relaxing even more ... you'll enjoy the feelings of relaxation that are coming over your whole body.

Other sounds and noises are fading away and you are listening only to my voice...

That relaxation is continuing to move through your whole body. You are relaxing from the top of your head to the tip of your toes...

You are continuing to relax and feel more at ease. You are sensing, feeling and imagining peacefulness, comfort, and calmness all through your system ... You are relaxing in a way that is just right for you...

Now take your left thumb and press it tightly against the index finger on your left hand ... You will notice the rest of your body relaxing even more now, and soon the thumb and finger on your left hand will relax and your finger and thumb will begin to move apart ... As the finger and thumb on your left hand relax, the finger and thumb holding the pen continue relaxing and the pen will soon slip from your hand and drop to the floor...

When the (pen or pencil, coin) drops from your fingers, you will move into an even deeper hypnotic state, and you will keep your eyes closed until I ask you to open them...

DIRECT GAZE METHOD

This process is the Direct Gaze Induction Technique. This is one of the most powerful techniques in any hypnotists arsenal, however it is also the most difficult to use because you have to have flawless self-assurance. If you show any doubt, hesitation, or fear, it will reflect in your eyes; your subject will read it. Thus it can obstruct their response.

"I *want you to fix your eyes right here*." Take the index finger of your right hand and bring it up under your right eye. When you're looking the subject in the eye, it is important for you not to blink. Narrow your eyes slightly, enough to keep your eyeballs from drying out. Time you're counting in response to what you see happening in the subject's eyes. If you don't see any response, stretch out the suggestions. (*Five eyelids heavy, droopy, drowsy and sleepy, your eyelids feel so heavy. Four your heavy lids begin to feel as though they're getting ready to close. Three ...*). The moment you see the subject beginning to blink, pick up the tempo and say *'And now they begin closing, closing ...'*

So now the induction

Now I want you to look right here. Don't take your eyes from mine. Don't move or speak or nod your head or say "uh-huh" unless I ask you to. I know that you hear and understand me just as you know it. If you follow my simple instructions, there is nothing in this world that can keep you from entering into a very deep and pleasant state of hypnosis, and doing it in just a fraction of a second. Now, take a deep breath and fill up your lungs. (Take a deep breath and take your right hand and move it in an upward motion in the air). Now exhale. (Bring hand down as they exhale) That's fine. Now a second and deeper breath. (Bring hand up) Exhale.

(Bring hand down) Relax. Now a third deep breath. (Bring hand up) Exhale. (Bring hand down)

(Raise your hand up over their head, about three feet in front of them, two feet above their head, pointing finger) *And now, I'm going to count from five down to one. As I do, your eyelids grow heavy, droopy, drowsy and sleepy. By the time I reach the count of one, they close right down and you go deep in hypnotic slumber. Deeper than ever before. All right, Five* (Start moving finger down) *Eyelids heavy, droopy, drowsy and sleepy. Four* (Moving finger down) *those heavy lids feel ready to close. Three* (Moving finger down) the *next time you blink that is hypnosis coming on you then. Two* (Moving finger down) *They begin closing, closing, closing, closing, closing, closing, closing, closing them, close them, close them.*

They're closing, closing, closing, closing... One

Place a hand behind subjects head at base of skull. Grasp subjects left arm at elbow. With a sudden forward pulling movement of the right hand, say) Sleep now.

ASSOCIATION METHOD

You can close your eyes now ... And begin breathing deeply and slowly ... Before you let go completely, and go into a deep hypnotic state, just let yourself listen carefully to everything I say to you ...

It's going to happen automatically ... So you don't need to think about that now ... And you will have no conscious control over what happens...

The muscles in and around your eyes will relax all by themselves as you continue breathing ... Easily and freely...

Without thinking about it, you will soon enter a deep, peaceful, hypnotic trance, without any effort ... There is nothing important for your conscious mind to do...

There is nothing really important except the activities of your subconscious mind ... And that can be just as automatic as dreaming ... And you know how easily you can forget your dreams when you awaken...

You are responding very well. Without noticing it, you have already altered your rate of breathing ... You are breathing much more easily and freely ... And you are revealing signs that indicate you are beginning to drift into a hypnotic trance...

You can really enjoy relaxing more and more, and your subconscious mind will listen to each word I say ... And it keeps becoming less important for you to consciously listen to my voice...

Your subconscious mind can hear even if I whisper...

You are continuing to drift into a more detached state as you examine privately in your own mind ... Secrets, feelings, sensations, and behaviours you didn't know you had ... At the same time, letting go completely ... Your own mind is solving that problem ... At your own pace ... Just as rapidly as it feels you are ready ...

You continue becoming more relaxed and comfortable as you sit there with your eyes closed...

As you experience that deepening comfort you don't have to move, or talk, or let anything bother you...

Your own inner mind can respond automatically to everything I tell you ... and you will be pleasantly surprised with your continuous progress...

You are getting much closer to a deep hypnotic trance ... And you are beginning to realize that you don't care whether or not you are going into a deep trance...

Being in this peaceful state enables you to experience the comfort of the hypnotic trance...

Being hypnotized is always a very enjoyable, very pleasant, calm, peaceful, completely relaxing experience...

It seems natural ... to include hypnosis in your future...

Every time I hypnotize you it keeps becoming more enjoyable, and you continue experiencing more benefits ... So you will really enjoy having me hypnotize you...

You will always enjoy the sensations ... Of comfort ... Of peacefulness ... Of calmness ... And all the other sensations that come automatically from this wonderful experience...

You will be really happy that you decided to have me hypnotize you ...as you continue experiencing progressive understanding on your part...

You are learning something about yourself ... You are developing your own techniques of therapy ... Without knowing you are developing them ...You can have it as a surprise sooner or later ... a very pleasant surprise ...

Imagine yourself in a place you like very much ... By a lake, or by the ocean ... Perhaps you are floating gently on a sailboat on a peaceful lake ... On a warm, summer day ... You are continuing to relax even more now ... And you continue becoming more comfortable ...

This is your own world that you like very much...

You are going to find that any time you want to spend a few minutes by yourself, relaxing, and feeling very comfortable and serene, you can automatically go back to this feeling you're experiencing now...

You can put yourself into this world anytime you like ... There are times when you will want this serene feeling ... And it is yours whenever you want it ...

Continue enjoying this pleasant experience as your subconscious mind is receiving everything I tell you ... And you will be pleased the way you automatically respond to everything I say.

THE CRYSTAL POOL INDUCTION

This is a well-known induction I have included purely because it is so popular. Chances are you will have come across this or variations of it in your hypnotic journey

"Take a deep, deep breath in and hold it for the count of five, now release it as slowly as possible". You will repeat this five times with your subject, "As you breathe in feel your tension and stress build up as if your breath was a magnet drawing them. Releasing each breath slowly and evenly, each time you release a breath you are evenly causing a feeling of calmness, serenity and peacefulness...relaxed, now...

Take another deep breath in, hold it for the count of five. Releasing each breath deliberately and evenly, as you release the air you are allowing even inviting a feeling of calmness, serenity and peacefulness...relaxed, now...

Take in another deep breath Releasing it slowly and evenly, you release the air from your lungs feeling of tranquil, serene and peaceful...relax deeper now...

Feel your body adjusting to that easy rhythm of breathing. You don't even have to pay attention to your body your body remembers the rhythm all on its own, just let go ...enjoy these sensations of absolute serenity and peace.

Now imagine a beautiful warm summers day, the perfect kind of day... you're standing in front of a pool a large crystal clear pool ... the cool air from the pool feeling so good as it passes over you, so soothing so relaxing as you watch the light sparkle and dance on the surface of the water... just across from the poll is a large weeping willow tree, it fronds reaching down just touching the surface of the water,... each gentle gust of air causing the leaves to just , gently, touch the surface making rings move outward all over the surface of the pond...

It would be so nice to step into this pool you want to feel the calm revitalizing water don't you? Take the first step into the water

you can feel the coolness envelop your foot. And now another step, sinking a little deeper into the pool ... the water moves past your ankles it feels so good to be in this water on this hot summer day. Taking another step now, lowering your legs into the cool refreshing water ... imagine you feel that cool liquid move around you helping you relax even more, it feels wonderful doesn't it?

Now take the next step down, standing waist deep now perhaps you can swish your arms through the water ... your whole lower body in the water, your eyes remaining entranced by the sparkling light dancing on the surface of the water. Glittering, so beautiful, in fact you now hardly remember why you came to this pool in the first place... now you do... to relax, to let go of the stresses of the day...

Just imagine how powerful those glittering lights must be if they can erase your memory... still your thoughts even for a few moments... Imagine how easily it would be for you to forget other things, worries, stresses limitations... all gone... Imagine how your mind is so strongly influenced by these dancing sparkles moving like little pulsed of energy over the surface of the water... did you forget for a moment that you were still in the pool... yet you remained relaxed... deep in thought... visualize how intense those sparkles are, and how they seem to be getting more vivid ... they fill your vision... imagine they are taking away any and all negative thoughts, negative thoughts are just fading away, disappearing

They fill your vision, blotting out everything else ... your eyes and mind filled with hypnotic, energetic, effervescent sparkles... there is no need for any other thought...

Everything else is gone and it makes you calm, relaxed, and totally serene ... with nothing but sparkles in your mind now... it makes you very relaxed wonderfully calm and all tension all anxiety just, drifting away... My words seem to be entering your mind from far away, travelling inward from far off ...into your mind and even though you don't need to actually listen, because you are so deeply relaxed, my words are embedding themselves deep inside your subconscious mind, going so deeper into your unconscious. Now there is no difference between my words and your thoughts.

From here continue into your scripting phase

RAPID HYPNOSIS TECHNIQUES

Being able to perform **rapid** or **instant hypnosis** is possibly the coolest thing in the world. However it does take a bag full of confidence combined with a lot of knowhow. Rather than make you undertake years of study, I will give you a few pointers that will increase the speed with which you place someone in trance.

First always set up the subject for future sessions, there are examples of this though the inductions, by giving the suggestions *"that you will fall deeper and more quickly more easily into trance each time I hypnotise you"*. You are creating a state of readiness, each time you work with this subject she or he will become easier to place into trance.

There are two important factors to consider when doing instant inductions. Firstly the actual act of hypnotising someone in the genuine sense, this takes a lot of skill you will need to select your subject very carefully. Making sure they are compliant, willing to allow it to happen.

Secondly creating the state we will call ***Direct Control***. Where... even though your subject is not entering hypnosis they act and behave as if they are, which then shifts them into hypnosis. You will be creating a ***Dual Reality*** situation where those watching, have a different interpretation of what's going on to those entering the state.

SPEED INDUCTION

Begin with subjects sitting in a straight back chair.

Are you ready to go into a hypnotic sleep? (Subject responds with 'Yes' here is an example of implied agreement or readiness)

Close your eyes and take in a few deep breaths and relax with each breath that you take. I am now picking up your right hand. (Pick up subjects hand as if you were going to shake hands)

In just a moment I am going to have you open your eyes and look at me. I will then count from three down to one. On the count of one your eyes will close again and your whole body will feel loose and limp. You will quickly enter a hypnotic sleep. Do you understand? (Wait for a nod or a yes signal)

Now, I want you to open your eyes and try to keep them open until I reach the number one.

Three, your eyes are feeling heavy, try to hold them open.

Two, almost there, on the count of one they may close and feel wonderful.

One, eyes closing and sleep.

At the moment that the eyes close firmly pull the right arm in a downward movement, reaching around and cradling the head forward as if placing them in a position of sleep deliver the command *sleep*, and whatever you do ...

DON'T STOP TALKING, go immediately into a deepening.

RAPID INDUCTION TWO

I would like you now, to take in three deep, easy breaths. As you exhale each time, I would like you to relax the muscles in, and around your eyes.

By the third breath you will have relaxed the muscles in, and around the eyes to the point that the eyes no longer want to open.

Now, take in three deep, easy breaths, and relax the eye muscles totally as you exhale. (The subject to take in three breaths, then proceed)

Good, you have now relaxed the eyes to the point that they no longer want to open. I would like you now to relax the eyes to the point that they will not open. Once you have relaxed them, make sure that they will not open. And sleep now At the moment that the eyes begin to shut down firmly, reach around cradling the head forward as if placing them in a position of sleep deliver the command *sleep*, whatever you do DON'T STOP TALKING, go immediately into your deepening

Sounds simple, it is, **with experience**, don't let that stop you from having a go at it.

THE OPENING LINE

Rapid inductions, believe it or not, work best with an audience. People watching tend to place the subject in a state of "I must perform or embarrass myself or the hypnotist". This why a dual reality situation is best used to induce the state. You can create a basic dual reality with a phrase that ensures cooperation. Taking into account the above examples of rapid induction you might want to add something akin to the following as you are getting the subject ready.

"Ok I'm about to do something a little different. So for the next few moments I need you to do everything I say exactly as I say it, and I promise you, you will go into hypnosis and you will enjoy it. So just follow my directions exactly, ok?"

THE EYES LOCKED RAPID INDUCTION.

Have the subject standing facing you.

Say the following or as close as you can paraphrase it.

Just close the eyes for me. That's good now just think about your eyes for a moment, and you know that you could if you really wanted to …if you really wanted to you could open your eyes

Wait for a yes.

But in a moment I want you to try and open your eyes

Ok now try to open your eyes

Good how does that feel?

Wait for a response

Good now just forget about your eyes

And try to open them…

Good how did that feel

Ok keep them closed now and just let all your body weight drop just let it become loose and limp and rest into me ok, that's good. Just let all your body weight rest onto me Ill support you. That's good ok… just let go and sleep now.

Your subject will lean forward where you can nurse them down or into a chair then move straight into your deepener.

Naturally this takes a bit of confidence, if you have ever seen anyone do it you'll be just as amazed as the subject.

The premise is simple you are causing fixation by standing in front of the subject. This causes them to look up slightly thus fatiguing the eyes, next you are employing the *Try Technique,*

These two principles working together make it difficult for the subject to open those eyes, the rest is pretty well easy to follow once you know the main principles involved.

HANDSHAKE INDUCTION

The instant handshake induction is a standard stage hypnotist's routine, it is rarely used in clinical hypnosis. However if you have the confidence and self-assuredness to use it, it remains one of the coolest inductions there is

Often you will see it being referred to as the Erickson Handshake Induction as it was developed by Milton Erickson, who as a student of hypnosis you are no doubt becoming very familiar with. This induction works along similar line to covert hypnosis. It is a perfect example of how to do a stealth instant induction.

You approach your subject (*this works better on someone you have already hypnotised in a past session*) looking for all the world as if you are going to shake hands, then suddenly as they go to complete the handshake you do something startling. The confusion principle with a **Pattern Interrupt**, causes their subconscious mind to be overwhelmed, the subject instantly obeys your command to go into hypnosis. Remember a confused mind will hook onto the very next thing that it does understand, in this case the command to sleep.

Erickson perfected the handshake induction during a time when medical science was still largely suspicious of hypnosis and hypnotists. Mumbo jumbo, voodoo and placebo they chanted.

Erickson was happy to demonstrate his handshake induction to these learned audience members during his lectures, especially those who declared that they couldn't be hypnotised. Erickson invited them to the stage. Offering them a broad friendly smile and his hand as they approached, they then plunged into trance dropping like a rag doll. These demonstrations of the handshake induction went a long way to convincing the modern medical profession that hypnosis did indeed have some merit and may even be a valuable treatment therapy.

So how's it work

As with other confusion or pattern interrupt inductions the handshake induction uses basic human reactions. People are more or less programmed to do things in predictable ways. From an evolutionary point of view this has helped us survive as a race, For example, when you are driving, you see a red light your foot robotically moves to the brake pedal. You never think about it, it is an automatic response. This reaction is so ingrained in us that many people do it when they are in the passenger's seat.

Once we have learned such routine behaviours they become unconscious or instinctive in short we stop thinking about them. This allows the brain to deal with other things that may be going on.

As a Hypnotist you are able to take advantage of these patterns. When your subject has some automatic behaviour pattern which they have performed thousands of times, they become locked into it, this means that once a pattern starts, the mind assumes the pattern will continue to its normal conclusion, the conscious mind stops paying attention, shifting into 'automatic pilot' However, if something occurs to interrupt the sequence of actions, then the mind has to stop what it is doing, focusing on the new or unusual set of actions that are now occurring. Conversely the mind will go into confusion trying to figure out what went wrong!

If, at virtually the same moment, as the mind is trying to focus on what is different, you were to start another pattern, now suddenly the mind has to switch again, paying attention to the new thing or set of circumstances, this leaves the first set of behaviours or pattern floating. If your second set of actions is unusual or unexpected then the mind is divided between thinking about completing the original set of actions and thinking about these new unexpected set of actions. It cannot do both at the same time.

No matter how clever you may think you are you cannot do this when you are surprised, when you weren't expecting it.

This causes a monetary, a few seconds at best, overload of the brain's attention function, the result is a few seconds of blankness. In that few seconds while the mind is in this state of blankness, it can be hijacked.

A sudden word or movement delivered at just the right moment during the blankness causes the mind subconscious to take control as the conscious mind tries to sort out what the hell is going on. During this state the mind will obey whatever instructions it gets, it is confused it wants to do something. The human mind also has a natural tendency to go with whatever seems easiest.

So how to do it

You approach someone you want to put into trance. They should not be expecting the handshake induction. As they get near you put out your right hand as if to meet them with a handshake.

Instead of going for the hand shake at the last moment move your hand forward to take their wrist, pull downward sharply as if to tip them forward and say SLEEP NOW... there should be a startled look on their face and they should blink At the same moment they blink reach up with your other hand gently covering the eyes keeping them shut. You must start talking immediately after you deliver the startle command. Just take a deep breath now and go deeper, let the breath relax you, taking you down deeper and deeper, relaxing into deep sleep now, go deeper and deeper ... as soon as it appears to be working take the subjects head cradling it against your shoulder as if comforting them and continue getting them to drift down and deeper. After the SLEEP NOW shock tactic do not rush your speech you will need to sound comforting caring and safe

All of the should have taken about five seconds this is maximum time you'll have before the subjects mind starts regaining control, a moment later they will start asking 'who the fuck are you ?'. If you speak immediately and continuously then most people will drop instantly into the hypnotic state.

THE MASTER INDUCTION

This induction deserves a special section of its own. Please go to the bonus section at the back of the book!

DEEPENERS

We have examined several things thus far, the process of convincing and testing, we have learned the principles of inducing the state of hypnosis, while very basic you should now be able to hypnotise a willing subject.

Somebody who wants to be hypnotised will be highly affected by the techniques and principles as you apply them. While you won't be able to walk down the street snapping people into trance, a willing subject however should slip easily and comfortably into state.

There are hundreds of inductions available in books, on the internet or through various courses, thus given the information that you have learned here you should soon be designing your own inductions, remember it is the principle behind the techniques that is important.

So having done this let's look at deepeners.

The idea behind the deepener is to take the level of trance to a stage where you can create effects, have the subject doing things , taking on roles or causing behaviour change, removing bad habits, fears, limitations, or allowing a fantasy to take over. More on this later for the moment we are going to get the subject into a deep state of hypnotic awareness.

Believe it or not the deepener is actually the easiest part, at the same time it is probably the most important, it is the easiest part because the subject is already in a state of hypnosis, and it is the most important because you need the subject as deep as possible if you are going to perform certain actions.

All deepeners work on the same principles, that of going deeper, you are bringing the subject down deeper. This is usually a visual kinetic combination of language that causes the subject to visualise a downward motion or sense.

You can use visual or mental idea that creates this sense, a stair case, an elevator, I've seen hypnotists use waterfalls ski slopes or anything else that the subject can relate to.

The idea is to go **down**... the human mind is preprogramed or hardwired to respond emotionally or psychologically to certain words such as **up** or **down**. So using words like **drop, down, lower** or **deep** can create a sense of relaxation and deepening.

STAIRCASE METHOD

In a moment I'm going to relax you more completely. Taking you deeper than you have ever been before, so just imagine for me now a staircase, with seven steps leading down, and because you are creating this staircase with the wonderful power of your imagination it can look and feel any way you want it to. There might be pictures on the wall. Carpet making each step soft and deep, but on one side... is a banister a railing that is strong and supportive, and will guide you on your journey down into deeper hypnotic sleep...

And you know that when we reach the bottom, you will be one hundred times as relaxed as you are now, one hundred times as comfortable ...serene ...and calm, and deeply soundly asleep...

Let's begin going down ...deeper and deeper down,

From this point on try to time the counting with the out breath of the subject so that each new lower number comes as they breathe out.

Seven...

Going down now deeper and deeper this is where every muscle relaxes and lets go of the last of tension, the last of anxiety...each muscle relaxes so,,, deeply,,, becoming heavier and heavier and there is a part of your mind that can quickly scan over you whole body... and if it finds any place that hasn't fully relaxed yet, it relaxes now... deeply... going down now deeper and deeper to ...

Six...

now that the body is fully relaxed ... this gives permission for the mind to relax... all negative thoughts just drift away... far away, it's like waking up on a beautiful morning ,high in the mountains,, looking out over the valley, and seeing other mountains in the distance... and just noticing the clouds that have gathered there in the night... and as you watch them, as the first warmth of the day comes in,, as the first morning breeze catches those clouds,, they begin to break up, fade away,, just like mist.. And taken away on the breeze far off toward the horizon... far... far away... out of mind ...out of sight... out of your awareness... that's how fear is leaving you now,, it's just breaking up and dispersing, that's how anxiety is leaving you now...just fading away, like a mist... that's how tension is leaving you now...it's just being taken away,, out of mind ...out of sight,,, far away from your awareness... as we go deeper now deeper and deeper down to

Five... deeper now deeper and more soundly relaxed, each breath taking you deeper and deeper down now to

Four ... Deeply relaxed now ... every sound you hear making you go deeper down,,, now deeper down now to

Three... so relaxed now... deeply, deeply relaxed, down to

Two... and this is where the minds can separate,, the conscious mind can have its own thoughts its own journey, think about whatever it wants to,, it doesn't matter you will simply let those thoughts drift through your mind and away,, you don't need to pay any attention to them at all... The subconscious mind come to the fore now... Listening... learning being aware of my suggestions as we go deeper and deeper now down further and further down to

One... and sleep... deep ...deeply, deeply asleep now ... deep in hypnotic sleep...

RELAXATION DEEPENER

Turn loose now, relax. Let a good, pleasant feeling come all across your body. Let every muscle and every nerve grow so loose and so limp and so relaxed. Arms limp now, just like a rag doll. That's good.

Now, send a pleasant wave of relaxation over your entire body, from the top of your head to the tips of your toes. Just let every muscle and nerve grow loose and limp and relaxed. You are feeling more relaxed with each easy breath that you take.

Droopy, drowsy and sleepy so calm and so relaxed. You're relaxing more with each easy beat of your heart ... with each easy breath that you take ... with each sound that you hear.

ANOTHER RELAXATION DEEPENER

Your arms are loose and limp, just like a rag doll. As I raise your hand, just let the entire weight hang limply in my fingers. And when I drop it, send a wave of relaxation all across your body. As you feel you hand touch your body, send that wave of relaxation from the top of your head all the way down to the very tips of your toes.

And as you do, you find that you double your previous level of relaxation.

Now, once again, with the other hand (Repeat with other hand)

You should now have a basic yet clear understanding of hypnosis. A working model of the steps needed to place somebody in trance, we will now deal with one of the intricacies of the art, getting your subject to wake up!

WAKING THE SUBJECT UP

As you progress through your study of hypnosis beyond the pages of this small book you will discover just as many ways of waking someone up or bringing them out of state (because they weren't really asleep, they were hypnotised) as there are of placing them in trance

The most popular method is to count up from five to one

Remembering that in many inductions we counted down to induce the trance, so to reverse it count back wards

I use the following wake up both onstage as well as in my clinical work

Ok that's very good you have done extremely well. In a moment I'm going to count back from five to one, when I reach one, and not before you will open your eyes and return to full awareness, you will open your eyes and feel refreshed and very relaxed, just as if you've had eight hours of really deep refreshing sleep, full of energy,

Five just become aware of your feet, feel that energy moving up through the ankles into the legs through the knees, up into the hips the stomach the chest feeling good and wonderful now

Four all the muscles of the face, that's good, now just become aware of where you are, the chair you're sitting in...

Three the temperature of the room ,,the sounds around us,, the sound of my voice, and just let all your internal rates return to normal fully aware, blood pressure coming out of sleep into wakefulness,, heart rate coming back up to that which is good for you,,

Two breaking through to the surface now feeling good feeling refreshed and wonderful and wide awake, now

One and open your eyes and re-join us here in the land of the awake.

THE POST HYPNOTIC STAGE
(Getting Them to Do Stuff)

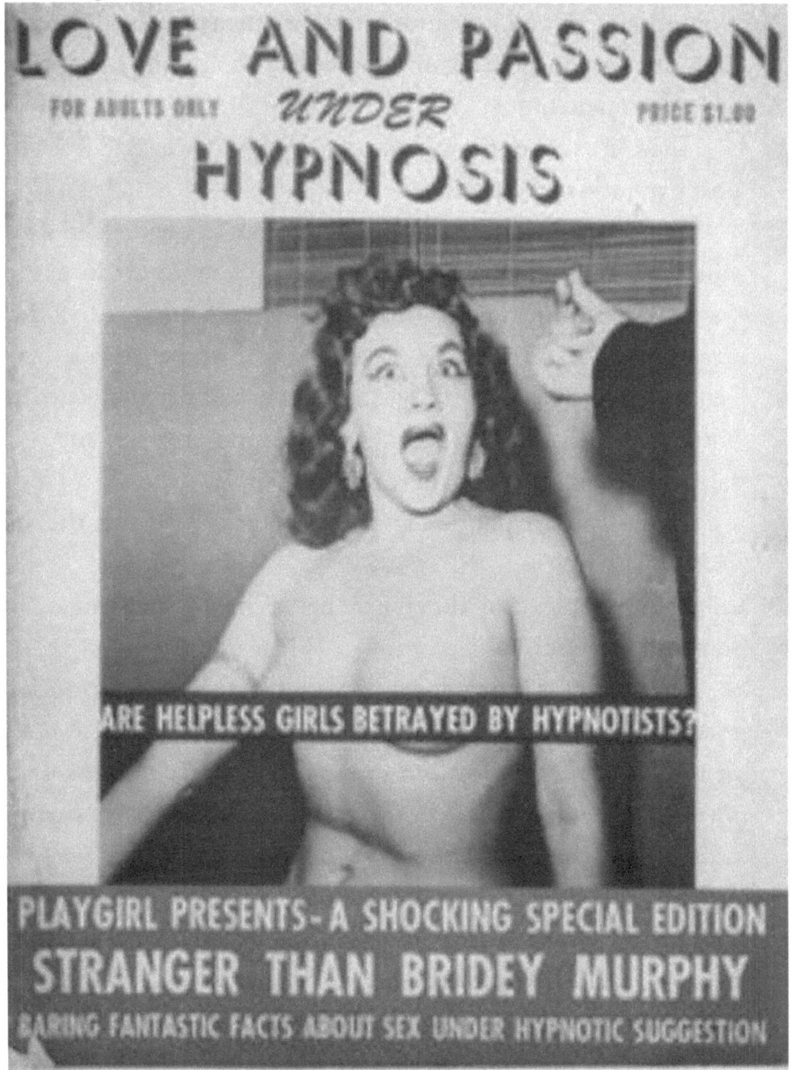

THE POST HYPNOTIC STAGE

So you have tested and convinced a willing subject that you can hypnotise them, you have induced trance then deepened that trance. They are standing, sitting or lying before you deeply hypnotised, so what do you do now?

There are two options you can perform trance state work or use post hypnotic suggestions.

Trance state work is getting the subject to believe things while still hypnotised, they will perform certain actions act in particular ways while still in trance. This is most commonly used in therapy situations. Where you are changing habits beliefs or harmful behaviours such as overeating, smoking or self-destructive patterns. Some of which can be applied to the erotic or sexual life of your subject. Getting over certain fears for example.

While a post hypnotic suggestion will take hold after the subject wakes up.

For example, the difference between the two might work something like this,

The subject is laying down on your hypnotic couch, you suggest that a feeling is coming over her, *a warm sensual feeling that begins in the pit of the tummy and grows like a warm liquid spreading through the body, this sensation becomes stronger and stronger, causing you to focus all your attention on it, on that warm feeling...and because you are focusing on it , it gets stronger an feels better, nicer more intense, focusing on this sensation makes it stronger and the stronger it gets the better it feels, and the better it feels the more you find yourself focusing on it, and the more you focus on it the more pleasurable it becomes,... it spreads throughout your body, as you focus on it,, it moves ... flows like a warm liquid down from the tummy up into the chest. The shoulders down into the legs so that it fills your whole body with warm liquid pleasure...*

The subject simply experiences these sensations revelling in the immense pleasure you are creating

A post hypnotic command would sound like this...

In a moment I'm going to count up from five...five to one when I reach one and not before you will be wide awake and fully alert, back to normal feeling refreshed , energised and wonderful . And when you wake up, when you open your eyes I'm going to show you an outfit, and this will be the most beautiful gorgeous outfit you have ever seen and when you see this costume you will think it's lovely, beautiful and you will see yourself in it, you'll be excited and imagine how nice and sexy you will feel wearing it, in fact this is the very outfit you have been looking for, for a long time, and finally you've found it, and its lovely, beautiful and very nice

Your imagination will run wild with all the possibilities as you see yourself wearing it, the compulsion to try it one will be wonderful and exciting and you will feel such a strong desire to possess it to own it to wear it that you will want to put it on, to feel it on your body to experience it, because you know you will look great in it feel great in it and be very desirable while you have it on, and you want to feel desirable ,,,don't you, yes,, so at the count of one you will open your eyes be fully aware and awake feeling wonderful

Then start your count out

Important things to keep in mind while using any post hypnotic suggestions is that *it must make sense*, the suggestion must be delivered in a believable fashion to the subject. Even if it is not exactly true it must sound true, for example you would not say when I wake you up you will walk over put this on and get Horny.

Next reinforce each suggestion as much as you are able without sounding nonsensical, three times is a good gauge, you can either repeat the suggestion or rephrase it three different ways or a combination of the two. Never give a suggestion just once, restate it, drilling it into the subconscious.

SIGNS OF TRANCE
How To Tell If It's All Working

How do you know if you're having an effect, getting the subject to trance out? There are several physical signs of trance that can be observed in all subjects. Of importance to you is the fact that a few of these signs cannot be simulated or faked by the subject. Which is a boon for your average stage hypnotist

There is always the fear that some yokel will fake it then spoil the show, however by knowing what to look for by being aware that the subject has no idea what these signs are, he or she cannot fake them. It is the same with the one on one session. Your subject will show at least one of these hypnotic signals you will actually be looking for more than one, you also need to be aware that some of them you may not be aware of until after the session. For example body warmth

Often you won't know until after your subject comes out of hypnosis how effective your session was. Many people report different effects during hypnosis. From the point of view of the hypnotist almost anything that is experienced can be considered correct, from the subject's point of view there are some common experiences. The most common of these are

BODY TEMPERATURE

Many subjects experience a distinct change in body temperature.

Which they can't tell you about until after the experience. They are unlikely to interrupt you in the middle of the session saying they feel really warm.

After the session Subjects may tell you that they felt cold, others will feel a sensation of warmth. This is attributed to the lower pulse rate with the extreme relaxation of the subject.

There are a few that you can spot during the session which will alert you to the fact that your subject is going under such as

R. E. M.

Virtually all subjects in trance exhibit a 'fluttering of eyelids'. The subject is actually in R. E. M. state. (Rapid Eye Movement) there is also eye movement or access, ask the subject to visualise or imagine something such as a tall tree, you may see the eyes move under the lids as they look up. Even though they are only imagining it, the eyes will respond, following the psychodynamic suggestions.

REDDENING OF THE EYES

At any time especially as you are doing the testing or convincer stage just casually observe the subjects eyes, there can often be a slight reddening around the edges. This is due to the relaxation of the muscles in the eyes which allows more blood to flow through the veins.

LACRIMATION

As they enter trance some subjects will have a slight 'tearing of the eyes.' This is due to the muscles surrounding the tear ducts relaxing

ROLLING BACK OF THE EYES

Entering trance will cause many subjects to roll their eyes back in their head. Simulating actual sleep, it can appear as if the subject is looking up, through the top of the head.

Finally the most popular cue for the budding hypnotist is *The Hypnotic Swallow*, usually occurring just as the subject goes into the first level of the hypnotic state, look for it as it is a definite clue that the subject is going under. The muscles of the throat relax causing the need to swallow. As the throat muscles are the hardest to relax, this is a very good sign that your subject is dropping into state.

TIME DISTORTION

The subject loses a real sense of time, a session may appear to have gone on for about an hour, whereas it only lasted for ten or fifteen minutes. The reverse can also occur, the subject opens their eyes then says "hey what happened that only took about five minutes, the subject is surprised when you show them your clock revealing that more than an hour has gone by.

Experience is a key factor here, as you practise on many people or get better at inducing the same subject you will see that subjects own little idiosyncratic cues. We all have them.

RECOGNISING DEPTH OF TRANCE
HYPNOIDAL (LIGHT) TRANCE

The first clue that you can even get to light trance is the amount of rapport you have with the subject, they must have a sense of safety, be comfortable in your company, your subject must trust you. This level is not too different from daydreaming. It will most often occur during the induction stage, before you have applied any deepening techniques. Your subject appears to be in a in a state just a little deeper than typical resting or relaxation. You should notice such things as a fluttering of the eyelids, an inability or apparent laziness to opening the eyes, reactions may be a fraction slower than usual. Breathing is deep and slow. There will be a noticeable relaxation with some sluggishness.

On the surface your subject will appear to be asleep, yet they will still be able to sit up, not fall out of the chair. Your subject will respond to any questions you ask they are able to follow any suggestions.

Another very good way of recognising this level of trance is, once you have worked with a subject two or three times they will be able to enter this level of trance almost as soon as you begin.

MEDIUM TRANCE

This level of hypnosis will most often occur during or just after your deepener, as the subject enters into a true hypnotic state. That's not to say that the previous level wasn't a true state, it's just that most of your "work" is done at this level.

While your subject is still be aware of their surroundings they are no longer compelled to respond to questions or suggestions. There may be slight hesitation in answering questions, or a sense of being too tired to actually do follow any suggestions. It is here that we use the pinch or other tests to determine how deep the subject is. This is where you will use scripts offering suggestions that take hold after the subject is bought out of state we will refer to this as the post hypnotic stage.

DEEP TRANCE (SOMNAMBULISM)

This is what you're aiming for. Sometimes called "sleep", self-awareness is gone. Even as you have the subject open their eyes, they are completely tranced out. It is at this level most of the hypnotic work takes place

PLENARY TRANCE (STUPOROUS)

This depth of trance is rare in the standard practice of hypnosis. Breathing with heart rate can drop off noticeably. The mind and body separate from conscious awareness. Your subject often losing awareness of time, body, or the external world.

TESTING DURING HYPNOSIS

On occasion it will be important to test that your subject is actually in a state of hypnosis. On stage this is done through compliance techniques, by progressively giving the subjects more things to do, or believe in. At first I might say you hear a sound or feel an itch, that's easy, nothing embarrassing about that, then I may give them something a little harder to do such as going fishing, driving an imaginary car or some other skit that involves more movement or stronger acting out or emersion in the belief,

Therapy is a different school. I need to know how deep my subject is, how far out of the conscious minds way the body, feelings or emotions are, so that I can talk directly to the subconscious.

There are various ways I can test this, I can use pain, by telling the subject that they won't feel a pinch or testing for full relaxation by lifting their hand watching it drop limply, fully relaxed back down to the couch or chair.

The relaxation and pinch tests are the two best, sticking a needle into someone is risky at best. Plus, I don't have a steriliser in my office.

THE PINCH TEST

Subject is relaxed you have just finished your deepener now you want to be sure they are properly hypnotised, so that you can begin giving suggestions

Say the following

Just resting now, deeply relaxed and very comfortable, in a moment I'm going to gently pinch the skin on your forearm, I will gently pull the skin up and give it a gentle but firm squeeze. (Place finger firmly on the arm so that the subject knows where to expect the pinch)

As I do this you will feel no discomfort, no pain, just an awareness that I'm doing it, (start a gentle pinch) *in fact like a gentle massage* (squeeze harder) *and a stretching of the skin you may even find it pleasurable, there will be no discomfort at all* (squeeze really hard) *just the sensation of pressure as I test your level and deepness of relaxation and sleep.* (Squeeze hard enough to wake them if they are faking or not hypnotised) *So just now taking the skin and gently squeezing,* (slowly release the pinch) *that's good you are deeply relaxed and that is fine...* (Let go of the subjects arm altogether) *going deeper now as I let go the arm resting falling back deeper and deeper heavier and heavier,*

A very important phrase is *"as I test your level and deepness of relaxation and sleep"* this subconsciously places impetus on the subject to *pass the test,* and of course the main idea of the test is that you are telling the subject that your squeeze will be gentle while actually squeezing them hard, a mainstay of hypnosis techniques is the *Altering Of Perception* as only a truly hypnotised individual will mentally *"read"* soft as hard, black as white and so on.

THE RAG DOLL TEST

Say as follows

Relaxed now deeply calmly and completely relaxed, so relaxed that when I lift your hand in a moment it will be heavy like a lead weight, like the arm of a rag doll, when I lift it you won't help me

at all, in fact you are so relaxed now that you don't want help me it will take far too much effort to use any energy at all,, you are that relaxed... your whole body like your arm is heavy limp, leaden, and when I release your arm it will drop back down with gravity it will just flop down like a rag dolls arm, and as it drops you will go deeper and deeper into sleep.

Now lift the subjects arm after a moment just drop it.

It should drop straight back down all floppy or loose like a rag doll. There should be no muscle tension at all. If it doesn't, if there is any hesitation, if they help you lift their arm, then they haven't relaxed all the muscles in the arm. Your subject is possibly anxious about the process which we will cover later.

In both case the pinch test or rag doll test, whatever happens is correct. If there is still some nervous tension or anxiety simply continues on, *"that's good relaxing deeper now"* adding more reassuring and deepening phrases as you go...

DETECTING PROBLEMATIC BEHAVIOUR IN A SUBJECT

This section is not really about hypnotherapy, or any therapy for that matter, it's about entertainment; nothing spoils entertainment like snags or hitches. So here are some pointers I've learned over the years from therapy that might help you enjoy the process more. Giving you a few strategies to employ if you come across an area that makes you unsure or things don't appear to be going the way you think they should.

Something I learned a long time ago was to observe a subjects behaviour, while in trance state, there are models of behaviour that you might expect plus those that you don't expect, the ones you don't expect are usually a good indication that something is up.

For example, if you are doing an age regression experience, either for therapy, as in discovering the cause of a problem, or for enjoyment, as in revisiting earlier exciting experiences for anchoring. You could reasonably expect a certain amount of playfulness or curiosity, if instead you get an outburst of temper, something might be up.

If during hypnotic *Age Play* your subject becomes overly dependent on you, once again something is up. Small amounts of these behaviours are perfectly Ok, but if your subject is exhibiting behaviour that would make you wonder about a real child, then you need to change tack or stop the play altogether talking the situation through. If you have built good rapport with a subject if know them very well these things should never occur. Because after all, the whole idea is to have fun.

However, let's look at a possible scenario that should cause you some concern (even though this may never actually happen) you are trying *Glove Anesthetise* on your subject. This is an effect where a hand is made numb then through hypnotic suggestion that numbness is transferred to another part of the body, such as the tooth during a toothache or the temple for a headache. In erotic hypnosis it could theoretically be used in many situations where control of pain or displeasure is needed.

The expected reaction is numbness with high insensitivity to pain. Perhaps during needle play or similar, the hand is numbed through hypnotism that numbness is transferred to the place where the needle is to go in. That area is now able to deal with the pain (or perceived pain) of the needle

Your subject shows this effect, but also seems to shut down on an emotional level, there is that extra sense there, a feeling or distinct impression that for the subject this shutting down has somehow included the emotions, that somewhere deep inside, perhaps subconsciously the subject has used the process to shut down painful emotions.

While this will be extremely rare I have no doubt that you will recognise it when you see it, nothing was said about "disassociation", or emotional numbing, yet the subject behaviour seems odd to you...

So watch closely observe how your subject behaves and acts, be in touch with their feelings their emotions, you will easily be able to detect anything untoward

ANCHORING
DEALING WITH AND ACTIVATING EMOTIONS

We all have Emotions; they are how we feel things. We feel them in our bodies as tingles or sensations such as hot spots, muscular tension even in some cases pain. Emotions can also translate as indistinct feelings like heaviness, cold or loneliness.

Emotions are cognitive, which means they occur in the brain, but are felt in the body, they are thoughts, yet they are felt as physical sensations, this makes them very useful in either hypnotherapy or erotic hypnosis.

When we associate with people or whenever we experience a pleasurable event, such as orgasm, we feel emotions.

Even thinking about certain people that we like or don't like, even imaginary people such as characters portrayed by actors, can fire off our emotions. By using anchoring techniques, you will be able to lock the positive emotions associated with good or desirable people or happy events to you. (The dominant)

Every time the anchor is activated your sub/slave/subject will feel positive emotions that they associate to whoever their favourite person is or relive those emotions felt when they recall a favourite or exciting event.

Anchoring by itself is a very powerful technique for change by adding the hypnotic state into the process it is made even more powerful plus it solves one of the problems that therapist have with basic NLP or cognitive anchoring, that being time.

While powerful, anchoring can wear off after some time, however by placing the subject in deep hypnosis any anchors you apply will last for a very long time.

From the point of view of the erotic hypnotist a very useful fact about emotional or sexual arousal is that there is a goal at stake somewhere. Our emotions cause us to want or not want. We are compelled to take some form of action to satisfy those emotions or desires, once we have achieved that goal or satisfied that desire, we then have a whole new set of emotions about owning it.

Emotions often lead to coping activities. The erotic hypnotist must remember that we move away from negative emotions, we strive toward positive or happy emotions, so when using anchoring techniques keep this in mind.

Each anchor you apply to your subject will have a result on their actions. When we feel something, we respond to that feeling. Sometimes this can be an immediate response, more often it is purely subconscious. You may not see it straight away. Even if you can't see it, there will be some internal change to your subject or submissives state of mind.

This doesn't mean that negative emotions are not useful especially for the master or dominant in controlling the slave or submissive. Where there has been a negative feeling anchored by the hypnotist / master, the slave's response can be anything from vigorous justification of the slave's actions to pleading apologies or other 'making up' activities.

Another reason we will use anchors is to aid the subject in controlling or being in charge of their own emotions. When we avoid or repress unwanted emotions it is sometimes a sad but true fact of human nature that we will displace those emotions onto something else. Often something or someone who doesn't really deserve that displacement. We act out our frustration in other ways. An employee pissed off with the boss at work may bring his troubles home to the wife.

Emotions are part of your submissives attitude or mood, our mood during the day might best be described as a more lasting emotional state. Each day our Moods affect our judgment, how we deal with other people or situations.

Another important reason we use anchoring is to deal with abreactions, as stated earlier there is no harm that can come from being hypnotized, however sometimes the trance state can bring up suppressed memories or darker emotions or feelings that need to be dealt with. Anchors allow the hypnotist to deal with any negative reactions in hypnosis in a calm reassuring manner, thus instilling confidence in the subject.

So managing emotions, both your own as well as your submissive, gives you greater personal control. In any situation where you feel your emotions may have let you down, such as when anger or fear made you lose an argument or made you say or do the wrong thing. Anchors can be highly useful always remember that the person who achieves their goal is often the person who has greatest emotional control.

ANCHORING THE "EROTIC" STATE

This exercise applies the process of anchoring, the conditions for creating a good effective anchor in either you for better emotional control or in a subject. We call this first state the "***Resource State***." What I hear you ask is a resource state it's the state or emotion, feeling or sense you want to recreate. For example, happiness, relaxation, or confidence, a resource state is a time in the past where you felt that emotion or sense of confidence then being able to access it now in the present.

Let's say you have a really important job interview, you are nervous, yet you know in the past you have been confident, it doesn't even have to be confidence at a past job interview, just a time in the past where you felt self-assured. The theory is that by accessing that past state you can carry it with you now into the present job interview, thus feeling confident right now

Accessing the resource state is best practiced in a location where you can be focused and undisturbed.

STEP 1

When working on yourself for better emotional control Choose ***a resourceful state*** you would like to experience more often such as self-confidence, lack of fear or being full of energy. Identify at least three specific times in your life that you fully experienced that state.

When working with a subject, submissive or slave choose the state that you want them to feel or experience, such as high sexual arousal, actual orgasm or that high point in *subspace*. The idea is to get them to mentally revisit the experience as closely as the can.

STEP 2

Have your submissive fully relive at least three experiences from the past where they have felt the state. Have them take a deep breath hold it for a second or two, then exhale, as they exhale tell them to close their eyes and relax associating themselves fully in their own point of view. Have them go back in time mentally to the best most intense time they can recall about the experience of that state. See the experience through your their eyes, ask them where they were when this occurred even if they can't or won't tell you, it's OK they can keep it in their own mind, have them *see* where they were, have them look around bringing in other details (*sub modalities*) have them recreate any sounds associated with each event *hear* through their own ears, then finally *feel* the sensations in your body.

Imagine your sub chooses to go back to their first really intense orgasm, reliving all the tension, nervous anxiety and pleasure of the experience. Your task is to guide them in fully remembering, mentally experiencing the event again, talk them through it, ask about *smells, sights, sounds*, make it as real for them as you can. Secondly you will be taking a mental inventory of the cognitive and behavioural patterns, both obvious and subtle, such as wry smiles creased eye brows, pursed lips etcetera associated with the relived experience of your submissive or slaves internal state:

You are helping them to listen to any sounds or words associated with the original experience.

You are guiding them to look through the mind's eye at scenes, details of objects and events which make up that original experience.

Get in touch with the sensations, both emotional and tactile, such as any smells or tastes related to the experience. Notice their body posture, breathing, etc.

Once you have finished guiding your submissive or subject through the experience almost reliving it. Noting their reactions each facial expressions the subtle body shifts and so forth. Stop them from thinking about the experience totally distract them shaking off the state. Start asking distracting questions like what did they have for lunch, how many angels fit on the head of a pin or tell them **not** to think of a blue elephant knitting a green jumper. The idea is to totally take the mind away from the experience, humour is a good way to do this.

STEP 3

Select a unique anchor. Identify some part of the upper body that is easy for you to touch, which is not usually touched during daily interactions.

For female slaves or submissives with long hair a good place to anchor is the line where the hair ends, where it just caresses, the back of the neck or shoulders, the first two knuckles of the hands, the knuckle of the ring finger, the ear lobe, or the skin in between your pointer finger and thumb. These are all unique areas of stimuli that will not usually be "tainted" by more random contacts.

Places that are not good for anchoring are places where we either touch ourselves regularly during the day without realizing it, such as the palms which get touched almost every time we interact with the world. The shoulders even your cheeks are often touched by yourself or others in the natural course of daily activity. Therefore, they do not usually make a unique enough point for an effective lasting anchor.

STEP 4

Begin to again to access the original experience. Watching your subject very carefully, look for that point where they are fully re-experiencing the state look for the highpoint of the experience As you feel that the state is about to reach its maximum intensity, firmly touch or squeeze the part of the body that you have chosen as your anchor. Adjust the pressure of your touch or tightness of your squeeze to match the degree of intensity of the feeling of the state.

After you have done this for a few seconds, as the subject is really getting into the state stop them thinking of the experience, shake off the state again. Distract the subject with some silly or humorous comment; remember the idea here is to make them momentarily forget about the state

STEP 5

Repeat 'Step 4' several times, each time enhancing the experience of the resource state by amplifying any sub modalities each time you install the anchor for example the first time you go through the process you might as you speak to the subject ask them to focus on colour, or movement, the second time ask them to focus their attention on brightness, to really concentrate on any sounds such as breathing or outside noises. as you perform the anchor each time you will be talking the subject through anything associated with the state, include as many modalities as your subject mentioned during step one, sight, sound, feeling, movement, smell and taste.

STEP 6

Test the anchor, have your subject clear their mind, relaxing a moment, for thirty seconds to a minute, chat about something completely disconnected from the subject at hand, as they chat simply reach out touching or squeezing your subjects anchor location. The associated experience of the original state should arise spontaneously without any conscious effort.

You might want to continue repeating steps 4 and 5 over a few days in a similar fashion to **Pavlov** or that used in *Operant Conditioning* until you have easy access to your slave's or submissives resource state.

Once fully induced (which can happen after the first session) all you need to do is identify some of those situations where you would like to have your slave or submissive feel those feelings where you want them to be in that state.

If you are doing the process while your subject is in a light trance state ask them to Imagine being in various situations or places, as you describe each situation touch your subject at the anchor point. This will help create automatic associations to each situation you make them visualize.

You may also wish to establish anchors for your subject for other states or experiences such as relaxation, creativity, motivation and so on.

For those who like a bit of science with their mystery, this process is the same embodied by all biofeedback systems: A resource state is chosen and identified. As the individual accesses that state he is given feedback for it by way of your stimulus in this case the tightness of the grip or the pressure of the touch.

More advanced versions can be activated with your voice or by intensity of colour even a light or by pure visualizations alone. The point here is that after a while the feedback stimulus and the target state become locked together in the mind of the subject. The stimulus becomes an anchor for the state.

EXTINGUISHING AN ANCHOR

A common question is, "How long does an anchor last?" This depends to how many of the conditions for anchoring it meets. An anchor made of an intense response, a unique stimulus, a well-timed association, which has been performed at the right place and stage can last a very long time. According to Pavlov, some of the conditioned reflexes of his dogs were only extinguished with the death of the animal.

This is especially true with negative anchors such as phobias, if a child is scared half to death by a spider or has a very bad experience at the dentist, those fears can stay with us most of our lives even long after we have forgotten the original experience. Positive anchors, if placed correctly can last just as long however. Sometimes it is useful to have a way of changing or "extinguishing" an anchor. NLP provides a number of ways to have more choices about automatic anchors.

If you ever want to reprogram or "get rid of" any anchors you have established, all you need to do is "collapse" the anchor with some other anchor or experience. For example, you could squeeze your slave's wrist at the same time you fire off some other anchor. Remember, though, that when you fire off the anchor you wish to reprogram it will influence any ongoing experience, so that when you are reprogramming yourself be sure to pick anchors, states or experiences that are of equal intensity and strength to the one you are changing.

If you wish to strengthen an anchor make sure you pick a stimulus that you can keep fairly autonomous something that won't be accidentally fired by somebody else.

AROUSAL SUGGESTIONS

Think about a long night in front of a roaring fire the two of you laying on a soft blanket just holding each other you smell her hair you feel its softness she caresses your arms feeling their strength, their protection you feel the heat of the fire see the flickering shadows dance on the wall, hear the cracking as another log settles into its place in the hearth. Now you listen to your partners breathing focus on it become aware of every breath almost sensing the beat of a heart what else can you feel. These are all sub modalities, they are very important in creating truly amazing hypnotic effects and post hypnotic commands.

A sub-modality is a part of visualization, an experience or memory that we tend to leave out in normal conversation, by inserting sub modalities into your hypnotic work you can create amazing effects plus experiences for your subjects.

Normally they are considered an exclusive part of NLP therapy or practice. Yet I started incorporating them into my work with weight loss with some anxiety clients, to great effect I have been using them ever since. I've found them to be a poignant even effective addition to my work, since using them my ratio of results in hypnotherapy has increased dramatically. While I lay no claims to inventing them I have will brag that I have become very adept at using them.

SUB MODALITIES ARE

Size, taste, smell, distance, sound, clarity, distance or anything else you can think of that helps the subject visualize, imagine, feel or experience what you are telling them or want them to experience. The temperature of the air in a room the colour of skin, or the walls how far or close something is, a rough or smooth surface texture.

For example in smoking cessation the therapist might use the smell of stale cigarettes to enhance the power of his or her suggestions then that smell is connected to clothing the breath, the hair, all this making for a very bad experience.

In erotic hypnosis you might describe the feel of rope, the bristly itchiness or roughness as it tightens against the flesh. The cold click of hand cuffs going on, or the burning of heat, the burn of ice (yes think about it ice feels like burning)

MIND F*CK NUMBER 2

Light a cigarette then blindfold someone now tell them you are going to place the burning end of the cigarette against their skin, switch the fag for some ice then press it against their skin they will believe that you have burned them.

Advertisers have been implementing sub modalities for years, possibly without the majority of people being aware. Observe commercials from the mindset of a hypnotist, you will make some interesting discoveries, for example how far away or close a product is placed or imaged can have a significant effect on how we feel about it. The most common sub modality used in advertising is the smile, we see happy end users of various products all cheerfully applying whatever it is to their lives then smiling about it!

Another good example is phobia work. Anyone with a phobia of snakes or spiders will tell you that they are only afraid of snakes or arachnids when they are in close proximity. We know that spiders are all over the place that in fact your average back yard can have thousands of them. Yet as long as they are far away they don't inspire any fear in the phobia sufferer. Distance is a sub modality.

A way I describe sub modalities to my clients or students is this, we all know when something is moving, but how fast is it moving? Is moving toward or away from you? Does it get bigger as it gets closer? Smaller as it moves further away. Can you still see this thing clearly as it moves far, far away? What happens when it moves really close blocking out the rest of your vision what colour is it? If it's close can you smell it? Can you feel the texture of the surface? All this and you might not even know what the object is...

In the erotic context you might want to use the smell of your subject's favourite aftershave or perfume, the soft feel of clothing, the tight hot feeling of leather. The heat of passion (temperature as a sub modality) all these describe things in a way that helps the subject visualize or experience the suggestions you are giving in a fundamentally more realistic way.

For example let's look at a standard hypnotic script for self-development. The opening part of a larger script. Then we will re-examine it in the context of the erotic. This with similar scripts can be found online plus easily found in many hypnosis books, it is what you do with it to make it your own that is important...

After a suitable Induction...

Starting to go on that inner journey ... taking yourself deeper and deeper into your internal self ... finding that place ... deep inside ... where there is peace ... and calm ... and tranquillity ... and you can be curious about this place ... you know that this is your safe place your place of tranquilly and safety. Your special place... and because you are creating this place with the incredible power of your imagination, it can look and feel any way you want it to,...there can be nothing here that you don't want,,, nothing you fear or dislike has any power to manifest here... and you can bring anything you do want, here.,,,. Can be here. All you have to do is make it so... and you become aware of something now ... something that you have only been partly aware of till now ... you are becoming aware that this place ... deep inside ... has been here for a long ... long ... time ... it's almost as if this place has always been here,,, there is a sense of recognition... just in the back of your awareness... just waiting for you to discover it...

as we arrive here we are greeted by the firm ground beneath our feet...firm ...solid...safe... and as we arrive here we are greeted by the most vibrant colours the colours of the sky and the flowers blues, greens yellows and there are some colours that we don't recognise... but they are beautiful and they are ours,...off in the distance we can hear a bird or and insect going about its business, and we have arrived here on the most beautiful of days,, not too hot not too cool the weather is perfect, ... light perfumes floating on the air, feeling gentle breeze on your skin

because this is your place created by your imagination I'm only going to place one or two things here, in this place... and as you look around yourself ... taking in the tranquillity of the scene ... being aware that this place has just the right kind of light for your needs ... you notice a small babbling brook ..A gentle stream, just flowing, ebbing away, moving through your place... You don't know or even care where it comes from... or where it goes...you are only concerned with it while it passes through your garden...

While powerful, the above script is a part of a standard one used by hypnotherapist to build self-esteem or alter self-image. Now let's look at the same script adjusted to make a subject more comfortable with their own internal sexuality. You might be using it to increase he self-worth or self-image of your partner because they have expressed unease in these areas when it comes to sexual relationships. To save time we will only deal with the first few parts of this script. A good exercise would be to take the above script completely rewriting it for your needs

After your Induction

Starting to go on that inner journey ... taking yourself deeper and deeper into your innermost self ... finding that place ... deep inside ... where there is peace ... and calm ... and tranquillity ... and you can be curious about this place ... you know that this is your safe place your place of tranquilly and safety. Your special place... and because you are creating this place with the incredible power of your imagination, it can look and feel any way you want it to,...there can be nothing here that you don't want,,, nothing you fear or dislike has any power to manifest here... and you can bring anything you do want, here.,,,. Can be here. All you have to do is make it so...

and you become aware of something now ... something that you have only been partly aware of ... till now ... you are becoming aware that this place ... deep inside ... has been here for a long ... long ... time ... it's almost as if this place this feeling... this knowing has always been here ... there is a sense of recognition... just in the back of your awareness... just waiting for you to discover it...

as we arrive here we are greeted by the firm ground beneath our feet...firm ...solid...safe... and as we arrive here we are greeted by the most vibrant colours the colours of the sky and the flowers blues, greens yellows and there are some colours that we don't recognise,, but they are beautiful and they are ours,...off in the distance we can hear a bird or and insect going about its business, and we have arrived here on the most beautiful of days,, not too hot not too cool the weather is perfect, ... light perfumes floating on the air, feeling gentle breeze on your skin

Because this is your place, created by your imagination I'm only going to place one or two things here, in this place... and as you look around yourself ... taking in the tranquillity of the scene ... being aware that this place is just perfect for all your needs... just take a few moments ... to explore...to feel...to sense... you will make yourself so at ease with this place ... that you will want to come back here...to this safe place. Your place ... time ... and time again...

You become aware ... that somewhere in this place ... deep in the garden ... there is a small babbling brook ... a gentle stream, just flowing, ebbing away, and moving through your garden... You don't know or even care where it comes from, or where it goes...you are only concerned with it while it passes through your garden...

The water seems to swell and ebb... in time with each breath,...You know that flowing water is the breath of the life ... that each breath is the life force of the cosmos within you ... a liquid flow a feeling of warmth.. and (sexual) energy...and you know that this sensation was already there inside you... even when you stirred this morning ...that it is the flow of life, the essence of our very being... you can easily remember when it first began to grow

How that liquid became heated, hot like lava and built... until somehow... It ignited, it became a spark of energy like flowing electricity that spark became part of you from that moment.... it became ...and continues as a nervous eager energy....

Well, I'm sure you have the idea, this is partly **metaphoric** allowing the subjects imagination to do most of the work, by not directly stating that it is **sexual heat** or energy the subjects imagination can and often will fill in the blanks

EROTIC HYPNOSIS INDUCTIONS
THE SCRIPTS

Everything you have read up to this point has been to get you step by step closer to being able to perform these scripts confidently. You should by now have a fairly good idea of how and why these scripts work. The idea behind this section is that each of the scripts can be adapted to your particular needs or the needs of your partner/ subject. For example a heroine script could be for any hero or heroine from wonder woman to black canary or in the case of a male partner batman, superman, whatever you like.

Each script is a guide to bigger better things, ideas or concepts limited only by your imagination.

Now that you are entering into the wonderful world of erotic hypnosis more fully there are a few things you will need to be aware of as you continue. I've said earlier that consent is tantamount to your success as a hypnotist. Therefore you will need the consent of anyone you hypnotise. Common sense and courtesy, you will also need to know what your subject wants from the session. Sit down have a long chat with them about their needs their fantasies or any desires they have.

Some people just want to get over basic fears, like anal, or doing it in public. Later you can deal with your own agendas or needs, wicked wishes or desires, but always start with what your subject wants or hopes to get from the experience. Not only is this polite it also helps to instil confidence and security in the subject, after all you are making it clear this is not all about you or your narcissistic needs... it's about them it's about what they want.

In fact to get what you want often requires helping the subject first for example using the stripper script is going to be a lot more effective if you have spent a session or two helping your subject feel good about themselves or have helped them loose weight or motivated them to go to the gym, a toned body looks better, feeling good fills your subject with enough confidence that there will be less hesitation or self-talk about not being a stripper, thus making the whole process easier.

YOUR FIRST EROTIC HYPNOSIS INDUCTION

Before moving to the *Post Hypnotic* section, now that you have a basic understanding of the how and why inductions work, we will examine a variety of erotic inductions. These work with all the principles taught thus far. Yet they are for consenting adults only. While the first induction is basic it is also a learning tool. You will recognise the command stages i.e. *Place Your Feet on the Floor*, the compliance stages *And at This Moment In Time...Nothing Matters...*with all the other areas we have discussed plus of course the erotic elements.

The command cum for me now would normally be considered a post hypnotic command, to be activated during the waking stage of your subjects daily activities, I use it here only as an example. Later we will examine more detailed scripts for getting rid of fear, overcoming obstacles to pleasure, body image, incorporating hypnosis into role play scenarios, with a host of others.

Following on with our idea of compliance, this first script is a simple one, a good way to introduce your subject to the idea of erotic hypnosis, without putting the subject under any undue pressure to perform. It can be very erotic even a turn on, yet at the same time is perfectly safe, your subject will learn to be secure in your presence, trusting that you are not going to make them do something really obscene, (*that comes later*)

Once you have learned it, make it your own, adjust it to fit your particular needs and circumstances. For example where it talks about a lover you might want to switch this up to become *you*. The idea is to keep the main principles in the context of the scene, if these principles are applied correctly almost any induction can be made effective.

To begin...

Sit the subject comfortably, on a couch or in a chair, dim the lights or make the room darker (bright lights won't help this) minimise background noises, perhaps some soft music... in short create a hypnotic atmosphere to work in.

Make yourself comfortable... with your feet flat on the floor...And rest your hands on your thighs... Rest your hands down...And gently allow the eyelids to close... that's good... now just begin to allow yourself to relax...Letting all your cares and uncertainties go... just for the moment let them drift away, because at this moment in time...Nothing matters...As you switch off your thoughts...And just allow this time for yourself...So that you can unwind completely...And as you begin to feel more and more relaxed...Letting go of any uncertainties or problems...That may have been on your mind today...And there is no need to fight any unwanted negative thoughts...just let them drift out of your mind you might want to use the old Zen technique of noticing those thoughts,...Just as easily as they came...

I would like you to take a couple deep breaths ...Slowly filling your lungs with fresh air...And as you exhale ...You will relax more and more...With every outbreath...And as you gently slow your breathing down...You begin to feel more and more relaxed...More and more comfortable...You will feel your whole body sinking into the couch/chair...And you will notice how relaxed your whole body has become...From the top of the head...To the very tips of your toes...

Your eyelids have become very heavy...they may tremor at this moment as they relax...As you let go of any tension in your body...And all the muscles in your jaw have become limp and relaxed... in fact every muscle in your face is becoming loose, limp and relaxed, your jaw drops down just a little...And your tongue resting gently...you are beginning to drift down deeper and deeper...

Feeling more and more relaxed with every word I speak... with each and every sound you hear, each thought you have is, helping you to relax more deeply, more soundly ... as this wave of relaxation spreads down through your neck down through the shoulders ... And all the way down your arms through the elbows, the wrists, to the very fingertips...You might feel a sensation in your hands...As your arms grow heavier... as heavy as lead ... relaxing deeply, soundly...And you soon become aware of a growing peaceful feeling somewhere inside...A feeling of calmness, contentment a feeling of serenity and just letting go, as you feel every muscle in your chest and abdomen...Become limp and relaxed...

Notice how all the muscles in your back are relaxing...Almost like a mental massage...And all the way down your spine...The muscles loosen and relax...And as you drift down deeper and deeper relaxed more soundly...deeply...you know that your nervous system is, right now, sending messages of deep relaxation to every muscle of your body the more you listen and allow yourself to relax the more those messages spread throughout your body, to every muscle, every sinew, every fibre...

Now make this wave of relaxation spread all the way down your legs...So that those legs become as heavy as lead, and every muscle in the legs becomes limp and relaxed...So that you are completely relaxed from the top of your head...To the tips of your toes...notice for a moment the outside world...Fading into the background... any sounds around you...Or in the distance...Will fade into the background...The only sound that will matter to you...Will be the sound of my voice...Which will continue to take you deeper and deeper...

As you breath, as you focus on your breath now ... You continue to let go of any negative thoughts or feelings...And Into a wonderful state of relaxation...And you may soon find that your mind begins to wander...And it doesn't matter where you drift...Where you go...My voice will go with you at all times...So that you will continue...To respond to me on an unconscious level...And in a few moments time...You will hear me say the word...Now...And when you hear me say the word...Now...All the unnecessary nervous tension will have gone out of your body...And your body...Will continue to sink down...Becoming more and more limp ...More and more relaxed...And comfortable...Just feel yourself sinking down into the couch/chair...Your head sinking down into the pillow...Becoming even more comfortable...Feeling completely at peace...And calm and contented...As you continue to drift down...Really enjoying this wonderful feeling of complete relaxation...And there may be times when...You will not be aware of your body...You won't be aware of your body at all...As you continue to go deeper and deeper relaxed...Deeper and deeper relaxed...

You begin a journey into your inner world...To that safe and special place, that only you can go to... for the moment let your place take the form of a garden, a beautiful garden. Clear, soft, secure... All your senses are experiencing this, you see, hear and feel. You see the beautiful colours of the flowers, the greens the blue sky... you can feel a warm gentle breeze , just touching your skin, cooling you making the perfect temperature... because this is your place, a place you are creating within your imagination, you are in control... your senses are enhanced by this place each of your five senses, is heightened, your sight, each colour, every hue some colours are bright clear and attractive ... every sound, is pleasant, in fact there could be a faint, distant music in the air, perhaps you can hear the wind... a bird or an insect, the sounds of life going on, just happening... your smell, taste, and touch are enhanced, heightened.

Because you are in charge of your garden, because it is a creation from within yourself just let your mind wonder, look around until you see one particular flower that stands out, that presents itself to you a little more than all the others. ... Perhaps you see a beautiful, bright, red rose in your garden now... Not fully blossomed yet, not opened fully, it wants to open, to expand fully it is just on the point of completely opening itself to the world. See the petals, deep red in colour. See the green brown stem ... the sharp thorns protruding now from the stem.

As you look, as you notice more, you will see there are small droplets of water resting on the petals. You can see this easily now, See the rose's wine-red colour growing, deeper, darker now ... slightly red, then deeper in colour changing to a light purple then a deeper fuller purple... Slowly in your mind's eye you see the dark purple now the rose has changed to a very deep beautiful shade of purple. ... It does this without even thinking about it very much at all.

A moment ago I mentioned music ... Think of some music now that you enjoy, music that you have used to relax... and as you do, you immediately find it so easy to remember, you hear it play so clearly in your mind now that you are compelled to focus on the sounds, the tones. The more you think about it, the better your mind can hear it now. It becomes very clear almost as if you can hear it, the more your body relaxes and your mind follows to the music without even trying to think about it... it just flows ...filling the background, it may be just out of your awareness ...but it is there....

Now using nothing but your imagination again, I want you to imagine a soft appealing smell in the air... you might be taking in the smell of the opposite sex, perhaps it is an alluring perfume. Possibly it is a soapy clean smell. ... Maybe it is the erotic smell of sex that wafts so easily in with each breath.

Allow the aroma to grow ... you can allow it to bring back memories, perhaps they are pleasant, seductive, maybe they are passionate, fiery, heated ... you are allowed to let those memories created by the sent to turn you on. You also notice that this happens very easily, very naturally... you feel excited by the idea that you can be aroused in such a way.

In fact, as the scent increases now, you find your arousal level grows with each sound you hear, remembering with each thought of the flower opening itself to the world, in fact every thought you have is becoming increasingly better ... and you find it easier and easier to just follow my words... to enjoy the feelings I am giving you now.

Actually you are not even wondering about anything at this moment, only the erotic aroma around you now. How it's effecting you, how it's making you feel it is like a wonderful exciting alluring hand guiding you and making you even more excited now.

Did you know that your sense of smell is directly affected by and because of your taste...? I suspect you did know this, its part of our natural life experience, that smell and taste work together, that they enhance each other... I want you to think of a sweet taste perhaps the taste of chocolate, whether it is, dark or white chocolate... Just think of the chocolate you enjoy now, and taste it as it enters your mouth, the texture as it first touched your tongue...

There is no need to think of anything but the delicious flavour... of the chocolate... as it melts on your tongue as it rolls around your mouth feel it touch the roof of your mouth, savouring the flavour, don't swallowing it, savour it. Enjoy the sensation the smell and taste as the portion in your mouth turns slowly from solid ... to liquid ... sliding like an ice cube melting in the sun. Feel a boost of energy and the first tingling's of erotic pleasure ... they are the result of such licentious chocolate. There was a time when chocolate was banned in many countries ... because of what you are experiencing now... there was a time when certain music was banned simply because of what your experiencing right now... a rush that fills your body ... your pulse quickens ... you want more and more.

Using your Imagination again just imagine that you can feel the presence of a lover...you have waited in heavy anticipation for their arrival. You have made yourself presentable for them. You look your best, you are clean you smell nice, just take in your personal aroma, you are ready...

Wanting ...waiting... excited. Feel their arms take you in, holding you in a warm embrace ... the first kiss comes ... soft and loving. It gives you such wonderful shudders all over your body, and for a moment you see the flower again... opening now... turning a deeper shade of red... and the kissing is heavier now... passionate, heated...

You can feel the heat of their breath and the warmth of their body pressed close to yours. You hear, whispering ... what are they saying...what are the words hear ... take in the tones and sound of the voice, breathy, passionate wanting. You must accept now that you are the vessel of this person's desire. The reason for their passion, their excitement... the heat...Feel your body so aroused now as a hand finds you ... touches you... this is a touch you crave now.

You can feel your need for more grow. You want... need more of this touch, the pressure of the hand , finding places on your body...The more you imagine this, the more you think about it, the more your arousal grows. In fact, this happens without any effort at all. It is just natural... perfectly natural to imagine to think about the smells the tastes the pressure of a gentle or firm touch and to grow more and more excited by these thoughts...for those thoughts to actually effect your body...to affect your whole being...for you to become those thoughts.

Each word, every sound, all the smells tastes and sensations you are feeling now are growing, becoming stronger, taking over ...

It is now possible for you to feel this way wherever you need to now, or whenever you are required to ... the sensation is so strong, so ingrained that you don't want it to go away. You love the sense of these thoughts, images Caressing your mind and body ... these feelings will make you desire them in reality, to long for, to seek out the feel of your lover's hands to let them explore your body. Let them touch you to excite you almost as if your entire body, as if your very skin is now your greatest sexual organ, there seems to be no part of you that cannot be excited by that touch... The more you feel, the more you want to feel. You crave more. Your sense of taste is also a sexual stimulant, your sense of smell is an arousal centre, and all these connect to your mind. Your imagination is a highly developed sexual organ... You need more and it is so easy to just let my voice guide you ... you find it easy to simply listen and allow yourself to let go of any inhibitions, any resistance just floats away with each word. In fact you want to follow each and every word as if my words were actually touching you... touching you where you need them to touch you now.

Follow my words and relax more and more deeply...sounder... going ten times deeper now.

Later you can add the following post hypnotic section to the induction. Do not pause o hesitate, just continue on as part of the same session.

and now just as you are enjoying my voice... and my words and the pleasure they are giving you, you will Crave the touch the feel of pressure on your skin, my words...even the sound of my voice is making you want more, ... the more you listen the more you seem to want... and You want the touch ... the feel of both softness and firmness on your flesh... You need the control, you have always desired it, both secretly and openly ... Just relax and let my words caress you now

relaxing 10 times deeper NOW...Letting my voice take you to a deep... deep state now A deep state of relaxation NOW and now A deep erotic sensation

The erotic pleasure is growing the deeper you go You want the sensual pleasure... go deeper and deeper now Letting the pleasure grow You feel the need to cum now You want to cum now And when I say the words "CUM NOW" You will begin to orgasm ... it is an orgasm so powerful that it will shake your very being ... so deep ... so intense that it will be felt throughout your entire body, every muscle will tense and harden becoming tight...as a part of you tries to fight it... but the rest of you wants it so badly that it builds ready to explode ... An orgasm so good That you will know it is the best orgasm of your life ... so powerful and so deep, you will feel the orgasm continue on This orgasm will last longer than ever before ... and then when you feel it begin to waver Another will take its place Even better than the last orgasm... The pressure will build consuming you until it also is ready to explode ... it will be as if every good orgasm you have ever had, as if every intense magical explosion you have ever experienced is returning ready to cum now...You feel the need to cum building now as if you can't wait for me to give you the command to cum, to allow you to release to build up, to release the pressure on your body and your mind... now You need to cum ... You want to cum ... the urgency is building ... The pleasure just continues to grow Deeper and deeper now, so willing to do as I tell you now, even if just to release the pressure ... Wanting to orgasm so badly You would do anything to have your orgasm and when you are done cuming, just as you think you are getting your breath back, just as you think it's over...there will be another... even more powerful, more intense, much deeper... You wish you could release that pressure, experience that pleasure now ... but you can't, you have to wait for me to allow it... to let you...

But you want to orgasm now you want to explode with pleasure you want me to allow it... You are so heated now You CRAVE release ... Once you are finished, you will thank me, this part of your pleasure, knowing that I am responsible or your pleasure, knowing that I allowed you to cum...

knowing the sound of my voice... my words knowing that my power over you did this to you when I say cum now you will release you will let go of the most powerful orgasm of your life ... 3...2...1... CUM NOW

SEXUAL ENHANCEMENT SCRIPT

The script used here is a commanding or instructional script (non-passive) remember the idea you are transmitting to your subject is that you are in charge, start and finish with this tone having the subject follow instructions rather than go along with your suggestions. This script also assumes that you have hypnotised this subject before, that they are somewhat skilled at entering the trance state.

Once again your subject is lying or sitting...

Now just relax by taking a deep breath for me ... that's good... and another deep breath, this time take in as much air as you can ... excellent now one last time take in a deep, deep breath and as you exhale this time just close your eyes for me... now starting at the top of your head just relax each and every muscle, relax the muscles of your scalp, your forehead, the eyes the cheek bones, moving down the face each muscle relaxing ... the tiny muscles around the mouth, even those muscles inside the mouth... down the neck, into the shoulders and down deeper and deeper to the chest and the tummy (stomach) relaxing through the hips then down deeper to the legs ... go deeper now deeper still let every breath you take, make you go deeper becoming more and more relaxed with each moment...

Now for a moment I want you to become aware of your senses, your senses will be heightened as you think about them, your sense of smell, touch, hearing, sight and as you think of them your senses become even more intensely heightened. Super sensitive and more noticeable perhaps even incredibly acute... your sense of smell is becoming heightened every breath of air is filled with energy, everything you smell reminds you of sexual pleasure, especially the smell of your partner (husband boyfriend wife girlfriend whatever is appropriate here)*, there is an eroticism in his/her smell, the smell of his/her body, his perfume aftershave reminds you of his touch.*

That small makes you long for that touch... every time you smell him or sense him you will begin to feel an energy rising within you, a high sexual energy... and it will increase with each moment, the more you sense his aroma the more you want him, the more you want that sexual energy to increase... before now you may never have thought of smell or aroma as heat...but now you do you can feel heat and sexual energy in every smell...

All of your senses are more acute. More tuned into your partner than ever before... you are totally in touch ... with your sense of touch, every fibre of your body has become finely attuned to his touch, every time he touches you a sense of energy shoots through your body, every caress sends waves of sexual energy though every part of your body, you can't help yourself from being turned on and sexually excited by his touch...his aroma the way he/she looks.

You are completely in touch with your entire body. Everything you see reminds you of the free sexual creature that you are, even your hearing has now become highly enhanced and aware, there are certain sounds that cause that energy to flow... every time you hear his voice it penetrates your body, exciting parts of you that will respond almost as if on their own, as if you have no control over how your body reacts... sounds good doesn't it, to be a sensual creature, to be able to see feel and hear every feeling...every sound... every smell... an you will notice how you can feel your body. Every touch causes you to begin day dreaming, seeing you and your partner fantasizing, imagining seeing full colour images in your mind... For you these are highly arousing bought on by the senses... even now you are finding the whole idea exciting and arousing...

Notice how you can feel every nerve in your body tingle with anticipation and excitement whenever you feel see hear or taste because now your sense of taste is enhanced as well, your taste is enhanced each bite of food becomes a succulent journey, you can savour each and every taste... combined with the aromas of your partner, wanting to kiss to explore with your mouth and taste, this increase your energy... your sexual state. So that whenever you eat or drink you will be reminded once again of the highly sexual creature that you really truly are... feel every nerve in your whole body reacting to each and every sense that you can experience with every neuron in your brain you can feel yourself begin to get excited. Feel your body begin to get ready as the excitement grows, whenever you see your partner you will feel your body become highly excited. Whenever you hear his voice you will know that every nerve in your body is getting ready to receive and please him... every touch will activate every neuron in your brain making you think, making you fantasize filling you with sexual energy... Your body has a mind of its own. Your sense now activated have a mind of their own... leaving you no choice but to react, to receive, to please and be pleased to find pleasure in every sense, every sound, every touch... Sending pleasure all throughout your body. Sexual energy and desire surging through your body... now as I count down from three to one you will find yourself fully awake fully alert and know that these suggestions have remained and will remain in your subconscious mind... where they will control your conscious waking life so that from this point on you are a highly enhanced sexual creature... your sense have been enhanced to the point where all you can think about all you can visualise is sex with your partner, you look forward to it, are excited by it and you want to see them now...

3 ...

2...

1 Wide awake now.

PTF SCRIPTING

One of the mainstays of any fantasy is role play, when we were children a combination of play fantasy and being somebody else made up a good amount of our mental time. To be a cowboy a policeman an astronaut, a princess or shop keeper. To take on the role a part of our mind believed we were the character we were portraying. This is why play is also an effective learning tool.

Even stoic kids who didn't actually play because they were too serious would imagine what it was like to be a doctor or a lawyer. Mental play is a form of visualization which moulded, shaped us into what we are today.

As adults it is more difficult to play, yet we all do it, we just keep quiet about it. We are a lot less prone to running around the back yard with a towel attached to our shoulders pretending to be superman. Girls still have dolls, they just don't have adventures with them, dress them up or arrange dates with Ken. Now the dolls are for collecting or just for looking at.

Many people yearn to be something else *even if only for a while*, to become better, faster, more masterly, more slave like, braver, weaker or whatever the fantasy is. These fantasy roles allow many people temporary release from the day to day grind, plus they keep the mind fresh, active and functioning.

Creating a ***Personal Transformation Fantasy*** for your partner is best done with post hypnotic suggestions. The process enables the subject to fully immerse themselves in the role of another character, this may be a character that is able to do things that the subject finds too difficult to do, because of shyness, self-image or guilt.

For example you might want to your subject to play at being a stripper, they themselves have said wouldn't it be cool to be a stripper. However due to self-perception issues (perhaps she is a little overweight) the subject just can't bring herself to take on the role. She is embarrassed, the role even though desirable feels awkward. If she can't believe the role then it's going to be less than real therefore not enjoyable for either of you. Perhaps the idea of playing the porn star sounds like it would be fun yet your partner hesitates they simply can't find it in themselves to play the role, creating a PTF may be the answer.

Creating a PTF uses concepts from NLP, modelling, lucid dreaming with Erickson hypnosis all woven together to create a believable active scenario for the subject.

The following example uses the porn star scenario. Once you have studied it, you can get creative, adapting the principles to your own needs, make it your own. This induction script assumes that you the hypnotist have put this same subject under before. This time they have asked you to help them create the fantasy of being a porn star.

Take a deep breath in and hold it to the count of five, then release it as slowly as possible, just like a long sigh ... As you let go, feel those shoulders relax, now take in another deep breath of air, as you breathe in feel your tension and stress build up as if your breath was a magnet for them. Now let it out so slowly and calmly, controlling it as it leaves your body ... ejecting all that bad energy, causing you to feel calm, relaxed, and wonderful. Take another deep breath in, hold it till five. You can allow your body to naturally adjust itself to that easy rhythm of breathing... You don't even have to pay attention... your body remembers the rhythm on its own, just allow it to happen, just let go and enjoy this sensation of total tranquillity and harmony.

Go deeper now ... deeper and sounder... relaxing as you have before, returning to that very natural state, relaxing deeper and deeper. Counting down now from ten to one. Knowing as always that when you reach the bottom, you will easily slip into deep hypnosis...

10. Heavier ... deeper 9, 8, deeper now deeper still

7, 6, 5 more relaxed now... so wonderfully deep and soundly relaxed

4, 3, that's good every sound is helping you to relax now every breath, every thought taking you deeper and deeper down

2...

1... just let go entering that deep hypnotic state once more...and coming back with me to your garden ... your safe place, of imagination, peace and tranquillity...your place of creativity, fantasy... once again we have arrived here on a beautiful warm summers day... it's to explore ... just to wander about, there is no particular aim to your wandering, your exploring, you just want to look around, see what's here...

As you journey deeper into your garden you know there is more to discover...more to learn ... just Imagine that as you journey deeper, that as you wander, aimlessly you find a large clear pool in your garden, you are just standing in front of this pool on this warm summer's day.

The air cools as it moves over the surface of the pool...then it reaches you, like a cool breeze, feeling so good as it moves over you, if you want you can find a comfortable place to sit... perhaps nature has provided the perfect place, a natural shaping of the earth to form the perfect, Place, to rest...soothing and relaxing as you sit, rest, relax and watch the light sparkle and dance on the water ... you want to wade into this wonderful pool of water don't you? You can, just let your feet drop into the water... feel the cool water envelop your foot. Cooling your toes... And now you can just let yourself go ... right now you are thinking how nice it would be to have a swim, to let your whole body slip into the water... how nice it would be to just sink deeper into the pool maybe you could just float... the sun on your face as the water supports you, you could just drift... float...

Lower your shins into the pool ... imagine that you feel that cool liquid coming up giving you relief from the warmness of the day, it feels wonderful doesn't it?

...

Now take a next step down, covering your calves and your whole lower body is in the water while your upper half remains fixated on the sparkling light on the water's surface. You can swish your hands around , through the water, you can watch the light dance as you do this... it's almost as if you can control the way the light moves and sparkles on the surface... your also making small waves and rings that move out and away from you...

The water shimmering, right now the scene is so pleasant that you barely remember why you came to this pool in the first place. Can you remember why you came here?

Just imagine how powerful the twinkling lights must be ... it can erase your memory, it can just make thoughts, fade away. I wonder how easily it could make you to forget other things ... just think how your mind is influenced by those reflections, as they dance and move across the surface of the water. They get stronger filling your vision ... filling your mind, other thoughts are disappearing ...fading away.

Just think of nothing but the lights moving on the water, you can try to think of something else, but it becomes hard, your mind has become so rested, so transfixed that it just seems like too much effort to hold any other thoughts ... even if they do come, it is only briefly and they fade away...they just drift in , then out of your awareness... nothing much is important, other than to watch, to observe the sun reflecting on the water... they fill your vision, blotting out everything else in sight Leaving your eyes and mind filled with these mesmerizing sparkles of light.

Just for a while you can be perfectly happy, with nothing but those reflections in your mind ... there is nothing to worry about, no concerns or issues to distract you, it makes you very happy and relaxed, peaceful about the only thing that makes it through is my voice, drifting into your mind, just let my voice and my words go deep inside you ... going so deep into your mind. There's no difference between my words and your thoughts is there... my words are your thoughts aren't they...

Just relaxing now deeper and deeper, now I'm going to arrange for you to do something that you have always wanted to do, to become an erotic movie star. An adult entertainer, You have wondered what it would be like to star in your own adult movie, to be an x rated performer... it possibly started as a bit of a fantasy, just a random thought every now and then... just a little bit of titillation. But now you are going to make that real... a reality for yourself, because with your imagination anything is possible...

You have appeared in many movies, with me as your co-star, did you know there are many triple x stars who only work with their partners. Yes you did know this didn't you, and you have always wanted to see and feel what it would be like to be in the adult entertainment industry. Well now you are and you have been for some time,

You have been working in the adult film industry for many years and you are a well-known star. You direct, write and act in your own movies, because you are one of the most creative directors in the industry,

Many years ago when you first started, and you can remember this, you were shy and unsure, yet today you are confident self-assured and creative, always coming up with new ideas and scenarios for your films, a true star...

Every sense you have tells you are good at what you do, and you enjoy what you do. Your mind is your greatest sexual organ...

The time has come to do what you've always wanted...

I want you to picture a scene in your mind. A film set, you can see all the lights, the cameras... And you are getting ready to perform, to act in a scene from a movie... it's an adult movie and you...are the star performer. You might also be the writer, producer and maker because you have done this before you've had a flash of inspiration for your next movie. You've actually been imagining it for a long time, rehearsing the scene in your imagination, and you already know that making an adult movie is every bit as challenging and demanding as any mainstream film ... so Before you start shooting, make sure the set is ready just look around make sure everything is in place. Where is your movie taking place, I know that your very creative, you won't think of just a bedroom or a lounge room...you have a specific scene in mind ... everything is ready to go. Set the temperature so that the scene is not too hot or too cold.

Make sure the Lighting is set and tested so that you don't lose energy when it's time to perform. Because you are a professional you make sure all cables hidden so that they are not visible on camera... Test the boom mic positioning so that it does not appear in the shots ... Make sure any props or toys that you imagine in your movie are where you need them now all the technical stuff has been done and is out of the way

You may decide on a single-scene that focuses on an intimate moment with just one or two actors, or perhaps just you alone. It could be that you own a secret web site and today you are creating a creating a scene for your viewers...

You are creating scene today ... in today's scene, you are lying back with your eyes closed when you begin to day dream about a very erotic situation. You can imagine the camera zooming in just slightly on your face... your expression shows that you want to know what it would be like to have someone caressing you, or just taking you ... You have thought about this often whenever you can think about it ... this is what your viewers want to see. And you can imagine all those men watching you, fantasising over you and about you... It makes you excited to think about that to see those men ...knowing that they are going to masturbate over your images and videos... you start to wonder then you realized how horny you are making yourself.

You begin to run your fingers over those sensitive nipples bringing them to attention as you continued to fantasize ... Your hand wanders down almost of its own volition... to your (be as descriptive as you need to be for your subject) *through the lips of your vagina, you are dreaming that someone else touching you. As the soft tender folds of your pussy give way to your fingers you feel very relaxed. Slowly and gently working two fingers inside ... giving you a wonderful sensation throughout your entire body.*

You love to make yourself cum and having an audience... knowing that unknown men are watching you is the biggest turn on of all. (Continue as needed or desired be descriptive use your imagination) *Lying in the chair you feel your body slowly return to normal, but your mind was still racing. Your fingers are not enough to satisfy you, you need more...*

So in a moment I'm going to count from five to one. At the count of one you will be fully awake, wide awake and returned to your normal waking state feeling fully refreshed, alert and wonderful...

Count out as in the waking part of your session.

5... moving back towards consciousness, knowing that every suggestion I gave you during this session was in a way, real for you, that your imagination is powerful that even though this was a fantasy session , that somewhere in your subconscious mind the journey has value... just becoming aware of your surroundings.

4... become aware of your feet, and toes, your legs, beginning to notice your breathing, as it returns to normal. Becoming wide awake now.

3... just notice the chair that you're sitting in, becoming aware of the sounds around you, the temperature of this room...

2... Beginning to break through to the surface now... all your internal functions returning to normal. Heart rate blood pressure all adjusting to that which is good and healthy for a wide awake fully alert person.

1... opening your eyes now...

The above script is a rewrite of one I have actually used for clients in the past, the following script is also a variation of an actual script. As with all the scripts presented in this book you should adapt them to your specific needs, each of the inductions, or deepeners and finer details of the script can be changed and altered to suit you and your subject. From this point on I will spare you the minute details of the scripts the psychology, the NLP and subtleties, such as confusion techniques or saying the same thing in different ways, as most of them will be obvious to the reader. Enjoy them, play with them alter them, learn from them.

I have tried to cover as many variations of areas and scripts as possible, if I've missed any here, they may appear in the next book.

FINDING THE INNER SUBMISSIVE

With subtle changes this script can be adapted to males. The script uses slight variations in *Behavioural Modification*. The script will also introduce you to the idea of *Conversational Hypnosis*. Even though the following induction is an advanced one, it is only so from the point of view of not having done it before, once you practise it, it like all inductions will become very natural.

Start with a casual conversational tone almost as if you were teaching your subject about hypnosis or explaining the finer details of the craft.

Ok just sit and relax now make yourself comfortable, good, just let those eyes close down now... did you know that all hypnosis is in reality self-hypnosis. If you Google it and you will get something like a million hits. You can't hypnotize someone against their will. You have to agree to it, you must allow yourself to be hypnotised, because in a sense you will actually be hypnotising yourself, I will just be a guide... making it easier for you to enter the state... it makes sense. If someone doesn't want to be hypnotized, they simply stop listening ... Every night, as you drift off into sleep, you move into the hypnotic state, this is why dreams can appear so real sometimes... in hypnosis that same heightened state can help you to focus your entire mind, both the conscious ... and the subconscious... thus making any suggestions you give yourself appear real to the unconscious mind... Or the subconscious.

As I said it's all about choosing to listen, so, therefore. If a person wanted to go into a hypnotic trance, all you would have to do is keep listening, because you want to, don't you...in fact you could think of this as a hypnotic induction ..., where by simply listening and allowing your body to relax... and the eyes to become heavy ... you would easily and comfortably take yourself into a hypnotic trance, you would just notice your breathing, and how relaxed you are... and then, just be resting the same way you do at night, you would drift into that state between sleep and awake, where you can visualise very powerfully...very easily...

And because you've been thinking that way you will find that those thoughts begin to arouse you ... filling you with thoughts of submission, a loss of inhibition a loss of control. Remember hypnosis is self-hypnosis and the choice to listen therefore you must have those feelings and those thoughts because you chose to keep listening ...You probably have thoughts of giving in to someone, or you remember... being turned on when you had to submit to an authority figure. You may have even sought out someone to take charge of you in the bedroom, and there are times when you got very aroused when your partner did so... it all starts very simply. Simply put, you just relax. Letting those thoughts and memories just float around in your mind... Hypnotic trance is very relaxing, and the more relaxed you are, the more those thoughts, feelings and memories come back to you... the more they come back the more you slip into trance.

Breath in deeply through your nose, hold it for a moment, then let it go, like a sigh, a deep end of the day sigh, where all your work is done, all your worries are gone... and you can just let go of the day and relax. Just letting your body wind down... Just thinking about your breathing.

Just breathe deeply and relax. There's no rush. You don't have to make your body relax, you simply have to listen to me, and you will relax naturally, just let my voice spontaneously relax you... going deeper and sounder now... think about your breathing, and listen and you will relax.

Ok now, just bring your attention to your arms and hands... that's good, now just make a tight fist , just placing a lot of tension in both hands for me now... and now let go, , let them go. Let your finger relax, the palms relax the wrists...relax, you can wonder about that, just how to relax your hands, and arms. The mind is a powerful thing. If you simply imagine the idea of relaxation, it will take place. If you imagine stress and tension seeping out of and away from your body, you become relaxed, it just, sort of occurs naturally ... doesn't it?

Your mind's eye is very powerful, so we'll be using that. Imagine your whole body starting to glow with a very soft colour, the glowing orange of a summer sunset. Imagine that glow warming your body and relaxing you even further. And then, imagine that glow to spreading. Very slowly, moving at its own pace growing to the rhythm of your breathing, each time you take another deep breathe, Imagine the glow spreading. Through your legs, up into the tummy, the chest, the shoulders, the face all throughout your body. Every breath relaxes you a little more, each breathe takes the glow higher up your body, and pulls you deeper towards trance. More deeply and soundly towards the hypnotic state.

Focusing on your breathing, in through your nose, ... out through your mouth... that pleasant glow moving throughout your body, feeling it relax every part of you, perhaps you are relaxing now more than you have relaxed in a long time, and listening to my voice letting every word I say take into even deeper, sounder relaxation, in fact every thought you have, every sound you hear is helping you to relax more and more deeply... Listening and letting the subconscious mind be led by those words.

Both your conscious mind and your subconscious mind are going deeper into hypnotic trance now, the more you listen, the deeper you go...

and you have chosen to listen, to listen to my suggestions... as you are aware hypnotic suggestions are suggestions you make to a person who is hypnotized. You could disregard a normal suggestion ... however unlike a normal suggestion, a hypnotic suggestion speaks to you at both the subconscious and conscious levels... once agreed to and listened to, hypnotic suggestions bypass certain parts of the mind and can't be ignored. And you already know this is true...don't you?

Your subconscious might enjoy something that the conscious mind is afraid of, or concerned about, our deepest wishes and desires lay within the subconscious mind... and your subconscious mind can react to suggestions that the conscious mind might hesitate to follow... your subconscious mind, that part of you where you really live, where you day dream and imagine can listen and react to any suggestions about things that it really wants...... but then you already knew this, didn't you?

In your subconscious world you are a submissive and as a submissive you can let your mind allow that part of you to be released, into the conscious part of your mind, into your awareness and into your being...body relaxing even more now... as you can pay close attention to my words, because my words are important to you as a submissive, listening closely to each and every word... taking in every suggestion.

In a moment I'm going to give you some suggestions, hypnotic suggestions... I may give you suggestions that will instantly help you descend into hypnotic trance ... it might be as simple as a word or phrase. So that the next time we are together and I hypnotise you, you will just slip into trance easily and fully... and I may give you suggestions that will make you feel aroused... or I may give you suggestions that tap into your deepest desires making you feel excited and fulfilled by being submissive, by letting that true part of your psyche go by unleashing it. Setting that part of you free...In fact even the very idea of those suggestions and how powerful they can be arouses you ... they could even take you to right the edge of orgasm... once you allow them to, by agreeing to listen to them... by agreeing to let them into your subconscious mind.

And I will give you suggestions that give me complete control of your body and mind. Suggestions that will bring out your deepest submissive desires and wishes, suggestions that will bring out your inner slave. Because being a slave is natural, it releases you from thought, from responsibility, from fear... all you have to do is obey, all you need to do is submit and everything else will fade away...However right now you are still relaxing... Still focused on your breathing, still focused on simply enjoying that relaxation ... still focusing on my words. Because Words can be very powerful...Going Deeper and deeper now.

When someone who is naturally submissive is hypnotized, words will bind themselves to the mind, holding you more securely than any rope... because they cannot be undone, once my suggestions enter your mind they become permanent, concrete, solid... at the same time they caress you softly, making you feel good, making you feel purpose ... and they do this because you want this to happen. Words can tell you what to think. After all you came here and you agreed to listen... didn't you, you agreed to allow those suggestions to enter your mind...because this is what you have always truly wanted... that's true isn't it...

Going Deeper and deeper now

As you go into deep trance, now you realise that as a submissive, as a slave you don't have to be worried or concerned about anything, anything at all... all you know is ... all you really know is hypnosis feels good. Submission feels good what you are experiencing right now feels very good. You love this feeling.

Going Deeper and deeper now

Listen and repeat these words. Repeat them back inside your mind, let them echo. Let them resonate with you... hypnosis feels good... Submission feels good what I am experiencing right now feels good... I love this feeling. There is nothing sexier than just allowing my brain to switch off, to let go...

And you know that it feels good to obey it feels good to be good...When you are hypnotized, you need to obey. Hypnotized people do as they are told, because it feels good to obey... because they have already agreed that this what they want...

Listen and repeat these words. Repeat them back inside your mind, Let them resonate within you ... it feels good to obey, it feels good to be good...When I am hypnotized, I need to obey. I love the feeling it gives me to obey... it is my natural state...Hypnotized people do as they are told, I am hypnotised, so I will obey ... because it feels good to obey...

You enjoy obeying me, don't you, we both know that's true... It brings you pleasure to simply listen along to my words, and being hypnotized by me is so very easy. You just have to think about what happened here now, and how it feels... the sound of my voice and how it relaxed you, how it distracted yet controlled your thoughts seemingly at the same time...your eyes will close again. Even imagining this helps you go into a deep trance, and the more you imagine it, the deeper you'll go each time.

You are a very good slave you know you are... and you will receive, many rewards for being the best slave you can be... top of these rewards will be the feelings you get from it. The feelings of pleasure and service you get from being obedient... every time I give you a command, it will fire off something in you, a sense of heightened pleasure, excitement sexual energy, simply obeying a command will bring you sexual pleasure... even anticipating a command from me will turn you on...

So I'm going to give a command now... you will obey because obedience equals pleasure, obedience is pleasure and pleasure is obedience, Begin touching yourself. Do it now! ... remember you are not pleasuring yourself for any type release you might normally get from this... you are simply obeying... that is where your pleasure comes from, the act of obeying is what brings you the pleasure the sexual excitement, the release...Obedience is pleasure and pleasure is obedience. The pleasure of obedience, and the pleasures of the flesh, are building now they are becoming one and the same working together as you feel and sense your body... The pleasure of obedience is sexual pleasure for you now...

As you bring yourself closer to orgasm, when you find yourself at the edge, ready to orgasm, as the pleasure increases and you feel as if you're going to lose control, remembered you want to obey me, obedience brings pleasure you must obey me, you need at your deepest level to submit to me, you will obey every command I give you...let these words resonate in you now repeat them in your mind as you feel the excitement building and the pleasure... I want to obey you. I must obey you. I will obey you. Listen to your own inner voice saying these things, that you have always wanted, these words release you from any responsibility... any fear... again and again, as you get closer. Listen to your own secret desires... and let those words become stronger each time you repeat them now... more and more powerful. Repeat those words to yourself just one more time ... I want to obey you... I must obey you... I will obey you... notice how important those words are to you.

Listen to yourself now... Your breathing has quickened, you can feel your voice wanting to cry out, holding back a deep sexual sigh... touching yourself in a way that makes you want to release a deep groan of primal passion and pleasure, let the sound of your own voice, the sound of your breathing... heighten your arousal... now you'll need to finish, you will need to cum... when I tell you to ... only when I tell you to, will you be allowed to cum... you are ready to cum, you want to cum, And you will cum, but only after I tell you that you can release. When you release you will cum very, very hard... Harder than you ever have before, after you have released you will wake up. You will remember everything... my suggestions will still resonate inside your mind.

You may cum now...

BODY IMAGE SCRIPT

More than one submissive (or people in general) have issues with body image, how they see themselves can often place barriers between what they desire, what they want to do in life, in the bedroom or in play. Body image is connected to self-worth and self-value, which taking into account you are working with a submissive or a slave, low self-image is part of their fantasy life. The idea of what other people think of us is a vital key here. Thus the following script is designed to help with these issues.

The induction is rapid it assumes you have been working with your subject for a while, that they are ready to go into trance. It could be thought of as one of the more advanced inductions. Some therapists refer to these types of inductions as ***permissive.***

There are two accepted styles of hypnosis, the ***Authoritarian*** or ***Direct Approach*** where the hypnotist 'directs' the client into state using a script. This clever amazing hypnotist will generally have a stock format for most of his clients.

The ***Permissive*** or ***Indirect Approach*** however attempts to employ everything that is present, including background noise, past experiences, room temperature, as well as the actual issue that your subject has arrived with.

With the authoritarian style the subjects experience is somewhat limited, they might be aware of the sensations of relaxation or conscious of the hypnotherapist's voice and not much else. Permissive techniques are based on the ideas of Milton Erickson who we have mentioned before. The approach is more effective for helping subject experience change in their lives. It is a powerful method of helping people utilise the hypnotic state to access their own inner resources. It is in effect giving them permission to achieve or change.

When you use the permissive style it often creates a heightened sensory awareness each session should be designed to suit your subject taking into account their individual way of changing state.

This has the added benefit of making them less resistance because you are using their own behaviours to enter trance.

Have your subject sit in a chair. Comfortable but not too comfortable you want them to be alert to a certain degree, rather than flopping all over the place.

Are you ready to go into a hypnotic sleep? (Subject responds with 'Yes' as you are setting up a *Yes Set* a series of agreements that will literally make them take themselves into state)

Now close your eyes, take in a few deep breaths and relax with each breath that you let go of.

I am now going to pick up your right hand. (Take subjects hand as if you were going to shake hands)

In just a moment I am going to have you open your eyes and look at me. I will then count down from three to one. On the count of one your eyes will close again and your whole body will become loose and limp. You will quickly enter a hypnotic sleep. Do you understand? (Wait the second yes)

Now, I want you to open your eyes and try to keep them open until I reach the count of one.

Three, (they open their eyes, stare into them for a brief moment then say) *even though your eyes are feeling heavy right now, try to keep them open.*

It might be enjoyable if we start with a satisfying deep breath... And you know how hypnosis works , don't you (third agreement) *that everything you experience, every single element of the experience... the sensation of your eyes, ... of your ears, the experience of your nostrils, the feeling of weight on your feet or the lightness in your fingers, anything you experience as you listen, even just the sound of my voice speaking, even without the words I am speaking, just the tone of it ... can help you to fall into a useful, interesting, perhaps even surprisingly deep trance. The nice thing about a trance, of course, is that it can occur moving about or still, waking or sleeping, writing or reading, listening or distracted.*

Now some people enjoy entering a hypnotic trance by experiencing a slight shift in their bodies ... in posture their breathing ... heart rate. Some people enjoy experiencing a trance by noticing the movement or even the stillness of their bodies, or the warmth or coolness of fingers or toes, or the pressure or lightness in feet and fingers... Some people really enjoy entering a trance by feeling the movement within their own bodies ... the steady rhythm of the heart ... the rise and fall of breathing... the sense of apparent motion and balance, and they enjoy being hypnotized by feeling more, and more in balance ... more warm or cool, more still or active.

Two ... And of course, as I speak, the relaxation can continue. You can continue to feel how nice it is to relax. To either concentrate or let the mind drift... I don't really know if you would prefer, to sit quietly while I speak with you, or to have your body make small adjustments that will help you feel comfortable. I don't really know, as I speak with you, whether you would like to listen with your eyes closed and your ears open, or whether you would prefer to listen with your eyes open and your ears closed. I don't really know, as I speak to you, whether your conscious mind would like to pay attention to the stuffiness of the room or to the sound of the beautiful birds singing outside. Nor do I really know in my conscious mind, or even in my unconscious mind, what your unconscious mind will do to benefit from this conversation. Almost there, on the count of one those eyes will close and feel wonderful.

One, eyes closing and sleep.

At the same moment their eyes shut, pull down firmly on the arm in a as you firmly delivering the command *sleep* if needed reach over tipping their head slightly forward as if emulating sleep. Then without missing a beat continue...

So, I just wonder what your mind will do to benefit from this conversation.

I don't really know whether that benefit will occur spontaneously and immediately as I speak with you now... or whether it will occur self-consciously later today or while you're having dinner tonight, nor even whether it will occur in the midst of a deep dream after you have fallen asleep tonight.

I know it will occur I just don't know when, that part is up to you...

I also don't know, consciously or unconsciously, how long your unconscious mind wishes to take to fully convince you that your difficulty with your image of yourself has been resolved to your own satisfaction. So just here...just now, we'll just have to wait, and wait, whether the conscious mind is open or closed, whether the subconscious mind is open or closed. Since we are here to explore your ideas about yourself, it might be nice if you make yourself comfortable enough, but not too comfortable, just comfortable enough to go deeper into the hypnotic state as you listen to me...

As you go deeper keep in mind be sure that anything helpful that you feel . . . that anything positive that is of importance to you, anything that you feel will help your situation or improve the way you feel about yourself and your image will be kept inside you for a while... and that if you hear anything that is not of use to you, that you do simply let it go...

So I was wondering how you might make yourself go deeper into trance...you may enjoy simply counting yourself through down into deeper trance as we have done before, if you want to go deeper now... starting with the number ten and counting to one, ten . . . and a deep breath . . . and nine . . . that's right . . . eight . . . seven . . . six . . . that's good you're doing really well at bringing yourself down deeper and deeper . . . and five now . . . and four . . . And perhaps you become even more deeply comfortable now... three . . .

two . . . and listen intently now... and take a deep breath. . . and one . . . . . .can you go deeper still minus one . . . minus two . . . . . . you can count down as deeply as you like... minus three You know there are people who really enjoy being hypnotized, they enjoy it in the same way they enjoy traveling to new and exciting places ... They enjoy the anticipation, the arrival, and the memories of that travel... the new things they learn from travel and from change... And they enjoy the curiosity, the excitement of riding those sensations into a deep absorbing hypnotic trance. Minus four... five...

(At this point let everything be still and quite for a few moments, just long enough for the subject to count a little lower into the negative numbers)

I believe and I know that you believe that from now on, it is possible for you to have a positive body image, from this very moment, or when your mind is ready, in ten minutes, or perhaps a little later, the time is up to you, you can change the way you see yourself... you can have a confident image of yourself and your body... you know what they say about people who live in the reality of their place in the world, in the reality of life... they say people who are able to survive difficulty, people who can and do rise above their problems, their false beliefs, people who are able to embrace challenge, and change, they say that those people have a lot of guts, as though courage were an emotion organized by the stomach and intestines... I suppose it's like the mind body connection... you will have heard people talking about that...so therefore It doesn't matter if your body is exactly where you would like it to be or not right now, it's about the courage, the guts to be where you are now and know that that's ok... that its ok because you can be better every day, that you can find the challenge and improve every day...whenever you look at yourself or think of your body image you can do it in a positive manner... Looking at your body in a positive manner will help you to feel good about yourself and to continue to progress towards the body image that you really want... we both know that you can choose to no longer think bad thoughts or say negative things about your body... that's the mind body connection... what you think about yourself and your body actually changes the physicality of your body and it also changes what other people think about you...

Your body is your temple. It is sacred property and you want the best for it. So from now on you think only positive thoughts and have positive feelings toward your body. You are happy, confident, and progressing towards making yourself the best you that you can be... that's how this mind body connection works, what you think creates your reality... and it's reflected in our everyday language. You'll hear people saying things like, they have a big heart as if love were an emotion generated by the muscle in the middle of the chest ... they have a lot of backbone as if truthfulness or uprightness were an emotion kept in the spine... keep your chin up, means to have hope, people who have a good head on their shoulders, or a good pair of hands are thought of as good, strong, and confident... so your language, your internal speech and thoughts can determine how you feel and look...how you see or imagine yourself directly effects what you feel and look like...so visualize yourself ... right now standing right in front of a full length mirror facing yourself ... visualize your body looking and feeling exactly as you would like to ... as if you had already attained your goals .... Imagine yourself wearing, the exact type clothing you would love to wear ... the exact style ... size... and colour ... realize that this person standing in front of you ... is you. You are this person ... this person is in you and you are in this person ...

You are allowed to feel good about yourself ... see yourself in front of you as the goal you ... knowing that every day you are coming closer and closer to that goal...You are on a journey to attain your goal but you appreciate that on any journey ... every step that you take is very important ... physical emotional and spiritual... what you think, what you say are all important parts of that journey...perhaps as important as the destination itself ... and from this moment on ... you can take each step in a confident, enthusiastic way ... having belief in yourself, a good self-image ... and continuing to move forward ... you are in control and you are positive about your appearance and your image. You are happy the way you feel you are confident ... so as soon as you are ready... as soon as you decide that this is what you want... simply accept it and move on...

BECOMING A ROBOT.

I will leave your sexual preference to you, I'm not here to judge anyone. Therefore, I will cover as many kinks, idiosyncrasies and fantasies as possible within the limited pages I have to work with.

This next script will help you turn the submissive into a sex robot. As always, this script will use a different induction a different style of deepener with various other hypnotic techniques all included to enhance your learning to aid your growing expertise in the craft.

One thing you may discover is that different inductions styles are more effective in different situations or vary according to the goal you are trying to achieve with your subject. For example, self-help issues are more effective in the permissive style because the subject is helping themselves so placing themselves in trance empowers them to make their own changes. Conversely if the end goal is something that gives you command or control over the subject then a more authoritative approach is best, you are in effect setting up a situation for control from the very beginning.

By now many of the inductions will start to look familiar perhaps even enough that you can create your own.

All you need to do right now is relax and listen. They say the mind is like a computer that each of us is not much more than a series of programs firing off, performing their actions, their duties the functions they were designed for. We each have many programs that dictate how we live... behave...and react to the world around us... so if you take a moment to think about it, you would have programs for negative behaviour as well as positive behaviour. There is a program that can make you tense, upset, angry, fearful...there are also programs that make you relaxed... comfortable, confident...

If you take a moment to think about it you'll notice a relaxing sensation in your feet. (Wait for them to briefly notice) That sensation is very relaxing, in fact the more attention you pay to it... the more it relaxes you... and it relaxes every muscle so you can just breathe and relax. So just allow that program to run... it helps to close the eyes and just let that program do its work...

so just Relax... breathe in ... and out.

Your feet relaxing so deeply ... completely.

Breathing in ... and out. Let them relax even more deeply...

So relaxed, breathing in ... out.

Nothing distracts you, you can fully focus on my voice... on my words, nothing else is important to you just for this moment...

except your feet relaxing, and now the consciousness of that relaxation increases ... moving upward, relaxing your legs.

Breathing in ... letting all the bad air out.

Relaxing deeper and sounder...

Every muscle in your legs and feet relaxing... calves, the thighs relaxing, the knees relaxing, paying special attention to each muscle relaxing as it works its way up toward the rest of your body...

Your legs and feet so relaxed now.

Breathing in ... and out...

Each breath relaxing you further and further, deeper and deeper

as your legs completely relax, the sensation moves upward through the tummy to your chest.

Every muscle completely deeply relaxed... notice your back muscles relaxing now... all then tendons, sinews in the spine tranquil, letting go...in fact you will find now that the more you focus on my words, the more relaxed you become. And the deeper you relax, the more you want to concentrate on my words.

Inhaling in ... exhaling out... letting go...very calm and peaceful now.

...So deeply relaxed.

Every muscle so completely... deeply soundly ... relaxed...

As the chest and all the other muscles relax, the sensation moves into your shoulders... your arms...

Each breath taking you sounder and deeper.

More and more deeply, completely relaxed.

Every muscle in your body relaxes.

Feeling the muscles in your back relax more and more.

So easy to listen.

So focused on my words.

So deeply relaxed.

All of the tension flowing out of your body, relaxing deeper and deeper.

Your whole body relaxing more and more.

Feeling any fear any apprehension and stress flowing away with each breath.

Deeper and deeper, sounder and sounder

More and more relaxed perhaps more deeply than you thought possible, more than you have ever been before. The muscles of the face becoming loose, limp letting go of any tension whatsoever ...

So deeply relaxed.

Every muscle relaxing further and further... and continuing to relax

Now that the body is relaxed and continuing to relax you can relax the mind... Your mind becomes more and more tired with each word you I say, with any sounds that you may hear... any other thoughts just seem to drift though your mind and away... you might notice them briefly as they pass through your awareness, as they float through your consciousness...but then they go... far, far away...

the mind, the thoughts so deeply relaxed.

So calm and peaceful.

So focused on my words...

Mind become tired as you listen my words, your conscious mind wants to sleep... while your subconscious will take over for your sleepy, drowsy consciousness mind.

So deeply relaxed...

I am now going to count down from 10 to 1, with each number I count, you will become 10 times deeper for me, and then when we reach the count of one, you will fully and completely drop into the lowest deepest level of hypnotic sleep

10 so calm and peaceful

9 so focused on my words

8

7

6 Every muscle so relaxed... relaxing deeper and deeper

5

4 So very deeply relaxed ... so deeply relaxed for me

3 so very deep for me.

2 Deeper and deeper as you follow my words

1 Descending down deeper than ever before and completely relaxed ... keep taking yourself deeper for me. Guide yourself down deeper 100 times deeper for me now. So relaxed and focused on my words. Feeling so good the deeper you go ... so deeply relaxed now...

and your subconscious mind is now open and receptive to the suggestions you hear whilst in this state of deep hypnotic sleep.

Just focus on my words focus on my suggestions and let them seep into your mind, let them become your reality... you can let your conscious mind drift wherever it wants to. But at the same time just to let your subconscious mind imagine, drift into another state of reality... Make it reality, each suggestion I give you becoming vivid in your mind...and while you are here, you are part of everything and everything a part of you...and you find it easy, so very easy to open your mind...to let go of any barriers, fears or apprehensions you used to have... and you accept everything I say fully and completely because your mind is now prepared and receptive to everything I am going to say to you ... and everything I say, will be accepted and acted upon by the subconscious mind

...reinforced...it will have a steadily increasing effect upon the way you think

...the way you feel...and the way you behave and the influence of these suggestions will continue to increase over the next few hours...

Imagine your mind is, as we said, a computer, there are programs that control each of your functions and reactions... and you always want to be a robot, it's a lot easier to be a mindless robot...no choices no decisions to make you just exist and obey. It's a lot easier, a lot more comfortable that way... even if you can only do it for a while even if only temporarily, it is better to experience it for a while... than not at all... this has always been a secret desire of yours and now it will be ...right now the hard drive of your mind...the software of your mental computer is being removed... the programming that drives your functions, your thoughts, your feelings is being wiped clean...ready for a reset... as a result of having it removed and made ready for new information, new programs a new upload... you have become completely motionless, now you are unable to move, perhaps this because your hard drive has emptied or perhaps it's because you are completely relaxed so relaxed that you can't move, either way it doesn't matter, almost as if your body is no longer under your control, you can try to move but you can't, You try to resist and fail, now slowly the programs in your mind begin to delete... ready to be replaced by new ones.. Your old thoughts vanish, Your mind becomes blank... everything except my words, everything except my suggestions, your body is completely relaxed, your mind empty and open... it is now void of any thought... any feeling... all emotions have gone... In you're the void inside head you are only aware of my voice, it breaks through the silence of your mind, like an undertone, you listen... you obey

your computer programming is beginning now, new information is temporarily uploading to your mind now ...You are a mindless entranced robot a automaton controlled by its master, all of your old thoughts and mind are gone ... replaced by new thoughts, the thoughts of your owner, you are an automaton, without thought or feeling, a device, a series of computer programs and functions controlled by your master, your owner, there are no thoughts, no fears no worries that can enter your mind... and you know that this feels so good and natural because everything else has deleted from the hard drive... the program is uploading now...now every time you hear the word (insert your trigger word here) *you will be instantly compelled to obey, you will have no control over this, because it is your deep subconscious mind that is pre-set to function in this way... you will become mindless, ready and willing to obey, to follow orders, to do your owners bidding. When you hear the word* (trigger) *you will transform into a brainless robotic slave because this is what you have always wanted to experience...*

when you hear the word (trigger) *you will become a robot, a drone programmed to obey, you exist to only serve, only to obey*

You are a robot Your robot nature is in control of you now and your programing is to be trained to obey to become a the perfect robot ... programmed to obey, you exist to only serve, only to obey... from now on whenever I say the words (trigger) *your computer mind will switch into drive, it will turn on you will turn into a mindless robot You will say your name, (say their name so that they hear the following command) followed by "activated"*

And whenever I and only I say " (NAME) deactivate" your human personality restarts...you will return to your normal waking state. However and always any new programming added by me while you are in robot mode is added, saved, and executed upon by the conscious mind... all suggestions given to you are added to your internal hard drive.. saved and kept for later use, and executed once again whenever I say the word (trigger) then without any action from your conscious mind the subconscious step out ... You instantly become mindless you will say your name then the word "activated" and become a robot the automatic software and programming taking over your internal and external functions, behaviours and thoughts... automaton controlled by its master, all of your old thoughts and mind will gone ... replaced by new thoughts, the thoughts placed in your programing, you are an automaton, an android with no thought or feeling, a device, a series of computer programs and functions controlled by your master, your owner, there are no thoughts, no fears no worries that can enter your mind... you will feel only peace comfort and the safety that comes from this state of mind...

You are a robot you are controlled... you comply with all of my instructions and input you have submitted my will, you have wanted this to happen and now you are letting it happen... You have no will, other than the pleasant feeling that comes from being a robot... a feeling a sense so pleasing, so comfortable that you find yourself needing to come back to it, to be a robot again and again ... As you lie still now with your mind fully reprogrammed

with your Robot programming complete you begin to sense your new truth, your new reality... and as I count upward from five to one you begin to awaken...

Now wake your subject in the usual manner.

GETTING CLEAR OF GUILT

It's not all just fun and games or being naughty, sometimes your subject needs clarity. They need to know that what they are doing is Ok. That's there is no need to carry a guilt complex about who or what we are. Guilt is that feeling of emotional anguish that tells us, either wrongly or rightly that what we are about to do, or what we have been fantasizing about doing, could in the eyes of some people be wrong, or might cause emotional spiritual or even physical harm to some other person.

We often underestimate the rather significant role this feeling of guilt can play in our daily lives. We have for centuries been socially programmed to act, behave in certain ways. In fact there are large portions of society who seem to get a kick out of making others feel guilty, (usually about the very things they themselves are doing behind closed doors.) One study found that if you add up all the moments you spend feeling even just a little guilty about things, it adds up to a pretty significant chunk of our time each day. It works out to roughly 5 hours a week of feeling really bad about ourselves.

Guilty feelings make it difficult to get what you want the feelings themselves can hold you back, even though you may have done nothing, the idea that you are even entertaining certain thoughts can make you feel like shit. Those feelings compete for our attention, over riding all our other thoughts. Other Studies have actually found that creativity is considerably poorer when someone is feeling guilty.

It can make your partner reluctant to let go, to be themselves to enjoy life. Even mild guilt can make a relatively normal creative person hesitant to embrace all that life has to offer. So with this in mind here is a script that will help your subject overcome their feelings of guilt and shame. Keeping in mind of course that guilt can be useful ... in small doses...

This script should only be used when there is no honest cause for the feelings of guilt. It should not be used when there is a very good reason the person should feel bad about things that they may have done. . When it became obvious that guilty feelings are deserved such as rape, murder, burning down an orphanage etc.

As always this script uses another induction and deepener adding to your overall education as a hypnotist. It also assumes that the subject has told you they feel awkward or *guilty* about the stuff you might be asking them to do...

This induction is professionally known as the seven plus or minus two method

Even though you are learning it through the medium of a guilt script it is especially good for the overly analytical or intellectual type subject. Those people who are apt to pull apart every little detail of what you are trying to achieve. It contains enough elements of confusion that it become almost impossible to resist, primarily because the analytical mind is redirected to think about what's happening it fails to notice what's really happening. It also works really well with subjects who find normal relaxation inductions hard to do. You will also recognise many of the hypnotic language patterns being employed in this script, such as the "**can you not**" pattern the "**and**" pattern along with a few others.

Once again sit or lay your subject down quietly...

Ok I want to talk to you today about these feelings you've been having, the ones you told me about, where you feel guilty for having your own ideas and thoughts... just take a moment and locate where in the body those feelings exist... (Wait for some response or description if the subject can't locate any area, ask them to imagine where it would be if they had to guess)

That's interesting, because guilt is often a method we use, internally, to protect our relationships. It occurs at the interpersonal level and it has its uses, it is an emotion that helps you

maintain good relations with others. In essence, guilt is like a signal that keeps going off in your head, and it will keep going off until we sort of do the right thing... like wishing a friend happy birthday or spending money on Christmas presents... so it sort of has purpose...

But it can also be really bad... Guilt can make you punish yourself and not for any good reason... do you remember the harry potter movies... (Wait for a response if the answer is no, find another example) remember Dobby the head-banging elf... how he kept punishing himself for stuff that others had done, or even for other people's thoughts... there is actually a human tendency for people to employ self-punishment in an effort to ward off those bad feelings of guilt and shame or I'm not good enough. However, it's not always ourselves we punish when we feel guilty... is it...

All right, just allow yourself to be as lazy as you want to be... listening quietly to the sound of my voice... and while you're listening quietly ... concentrating for a few moments on that spot in your body where you keep the guilt... and just ask yourself, is that feeling real, or is it just a feeling I have... and while you're observing that spot... just quietly concentrate on your breathing... breathing slowly and steadily, and just let your eyes close down, just as if you were sound asleep, or pretending to be sound asleep... and imagining, just how comfortable you might look while you're relaxing in the chair... using the power of your mind to see yourself, in your mind's eye... and then using the power of your imagination to do whatever you need to do, to make that image look even more relaxed... and comfortable... and still thinking about your breathing, making quite sure that each breath in lasts the same length of time as the last breath in... and each breath outwards lasts the same length of time as the last breath out... even though each breath in will probably be slightly shorter than each breath out... and while you're thinking about your breathing, and still aware of that place in your body where you keep the guilt or those *bad feelings, or indeed any bad feelings... you might also notice, the weight of your head against the back of the chair... and still listening quietly to the sound of my voice...And while you're listening quietly to the sound of my voice ... you might become aware that you've forgotten to think about your breathing... but that's all right, you can just simply start thinking about your breathing again while you're listening quietly to the sound of my voice and what I'm saying to you here... and in psychology, there's a rule called... seven plus or minus two... this means that most people can think of seven things all at once... plus or minus two... so you should be able to think of at least five things all at the same time... the sound of my voice... the steadiness of your breathing... the part of your body.. the weight of your head against the back of the chair... and don't forget how you look from the outside...what you are doing to make yourself look even more relaxed... and that's five things... so you can think of those things while you're listening to any sounds that might happen outside this room ... so that's six things, now... that you can be are of all at the same time. Or perhaps your mind is rapidly sorting through each one of them, so rapidly that it seems as if your thinking about them all at the same time...and I wonder if you can think about all those things and then at the same time notice the way your feet feel on the floor... and perhaps how your arms feel... and that's seven things now... the sound of my voice... the weight of your head against the back of the chair... that place in your body... the way you look while you're relaxing... and your breathing... and your arms... and your feet resting... and I wonder if you can now add an eighth thing into all of that... I wonder if your mind is powerful enough to think of seven plus one other thing... adding in, perhaps, an awareness of the temperature of the room... and then just testing to see whether you can add yet another input to your senses... so that you're thinking of NINE things all at once... that's seven plus two... thinking about all those eight inputs to your senses and then maybe adding an awareness of the way your eyes feel while you're thinking about all those other things... the weight of your head... your breathing... the place in your body... how you look from the outside... the temperature of the room... your feet on the footrest... your arms... the sound of my voice... and how your eyes feel...*

The weight of your head... your breathing... how you look from the outside... the temperature of the room... your feet on the footrest... your arms... the sound of my voice... and how your eyes feel... and of course, when anybody thinks of all these things, what they are really doing is scanning round them one after the other... very quickly... so quickly, it feels as if you're thinking of them all at once... and in the world of computers, that would be called timesharing... sharing your available resources between the different tasks you are attempting to perform all at once... and that's why some people can think of only five things... because it's the limit of their memory... while others can actually think of nine things... and I wonder how well your memory is working as you struggle to remember those nine things... the weight of your head... your breathing... the music in the background... how you look from the outside... the temperature of the room... your arms... the sound of my voice... and how your eyes feel...

And now you can think how good it will feel... when you simply allow yourself to let go of all that, to think of only the one most important thing of all right now... concentrating all your energies onto that one most important thought of all... which is going to be so easy to think of, now that you are going to let go of all those other extraneous thoughts, and allow yourself to think of only one thing instead of many... and that one thing is how good it feels to think of only one thing... thinking how relaxed you can be right now... only thinking of how relaxed you would like to be... relaxing in your mind... and in your body... no need to think anything at all, really... just let every thought go, no need to do anything... nobody wanting anything and nobody expecting anything of you for the next few minutes... and absolutely nothing whatsoever for you to do except to... relax.

Did you notice how easy that was, how easy it was to let all that go and just focus on one thing... you probably notice the feeling in your body shifted away as well. And you're going to find it just as easy to forgive yourself for things you "feel" (emphasise the word FEEL) *you may have done wrong in the past...whether those wrongs are real or just feelings, vague ideas of guilt and shame put into your head by society or other people's values and ideas, which as we know, usually turn out to be wrong anyway, they are opinions, not facts... and whether they are in your conscious mind or buried within the subconscious... you're going to find yourself easily able to let go of any guilt feelings associated with these things... this is going to be just as easy as letting go of all those thoughts I asked you to concentrate on earlier, because you are a normal human being, you have normal emotions and normal drives, you're sometimes prone to make normal human errors, as we all do... but those errors, those human mistakes, are in the past now... and the past is done, it is over and we cannot and we should not attempt to change history... in fact no amount of thinking about it brooding on it, wishing it could be different...can ever change anything that occurred in the past...*

everything that happened to you is part of what makes you human... part of the fundamental nature of you and what makes you the you that you are and the very fact that you are able to feel guilt tells you that you are human... it tells you that that you are a caring person... because if we did not experience guilt, then that would mean that we did not care... and it is only the person who does not care that should feel guilt... and yet it is only the person who cares who does feel guilt. It is only the person who genuinely cares, that does feel guilt... so now it's time for you to be just a little kinder to yourself...

you can now accept that the guilt you were feeling, is the subconscious mind's way of letting you punish yourself for things you feel you may have done wrong... which in reality, if you take a moment to think about it, is really somebody else's idea of what they think you should live up to, a false standard, somebody else's standards, values or ideas of what you should be like as a person... that's if you really think about it... there are times and places where a little sense of guilt is good, it can make us do the right thing, but 99 percent of the time it is nothing more than cleverly disguised emotional blackmail placed on us by other people... other people can make us feel bad or immoral, yet morals are subjective, personal values ... and history continuously shows us that morals change, what was wrong yesterday is perfectly acceptable today...

therefore isn't there a limit to the amount of punishment that we need to place on ourselves for any perceived wrong doing... every caring person knows that... that's why we forgive others...isn't it...and when that limit has been reached, there is no justifiable need or cause for the punishment to continue... is there? ... And a caring person finds it easy to forgive others their mistakes... don't they? ... And so now you can forgive yourself... can't you?

can you not forgive others for their errors, their mistakes... because those things you feel they may have done wrong were errors... just mistakes... so there is no need now for any further punishment... so now you can forgive yourself... can you not?

most of the time, nearly all of the time, you don't make these errors... nearly all the time, you do the right thing... and you have always tried to do what you believed was the right thing to do... and because of this, you're going to find it easy to forgive yourself, right now, right this minute... you're going to find yourself easily able to let go of any guilt feelings associated with these things that you feel you may have done wrong...

Whether those feelings are in the conscious mind or buried within the depths of the subconscious... it's all right to let go of those feelings of guilt... and to accept that you are a whole, complete, and worthwhile person...

Wake the subject as per normal

GETTING CREATIVE IN THE BEDROOM

Going to unexpected places.

It is now time for us to get a little more advanced. The following script can be altered or adjusted to many needs such as fear, phobias, overcoming bad habits with a variety of other applications. All you need to do is reconstruct the scripting section to suit your needs. It will become obvious how this works as you read the script. It also employs an advanced deepening techniques. Not advanced in the sense that you have to be super-duper intelligent or have years of training to use it, advanced in the way it deals with the human mind it creates a very, very deep trance state. Advanced in the fact that you will not have used or understood the potency of such techniques just yet.

To start with you are (describe where they are on a bed or in a chair) *it is a quiet place, free of interruptions ... notice your body begin to sink into the bed / chair and feel yourself become comfortable... Letting your muscles shift and move as make yourself and start to relax*

for the next twenty minutes or so, this is your time, no one else's, you can rest, relax and enjoy this time. Any apprehensions can be set aside. If they are important, you can go back to once this time for recreating your life has finished. In fact this time may allow your mind to find new ideas and new solutions to those problems, or at the very least new ways of thinking about them, change your attitude toward them... making them seem very trivial when compared to the rest of the world... and of course any important, that is truly important tasks, will still be there later.

As your body relaxes into its most comfy position, just you let the eyes gently close down... The muscles in and around your eyelids are the most sensitive in the body ... they are the quickest to relax ... as you listen, and as you focus on them you will notice that your eyelids get heavy, as if they are being held shut like those times when you are so tired you just can't keep them open, even if you try, it's as if trying to keep them open tires them out even more....... and as this is your time, your eyes simply won't feel the need to open again, not until your relaxation time is finished and you know that it's time to open them once more... in fact you are already beginning to experience a feeling of mental and physical relaxation ...

Now just let the mind wander a moment imagine a very beautiful private place on a dreamily brilliant day, the perfect day.... It doesn't matter if this is a place you actually know or of your imagining it, simply visualising or making it up in your mind, the fact is ... let's assume for a moment that this special private place is a garden... If you can imagine it, then it is real for you ... picture or imagine that as we arrive in this garden, you can feel the solid ground beneath your feet... notice that it is supporting you, that it is solid and firm... perhaps you can feel a softer moss covering the ground, it is cushioning each step you take.. ... it could be that you can hear the sound of some birds off in the distance... or the buzzing of an insect as it go about the business of tending to the growth and pollination of the flowers in your garden... imagine the smell of those flowers, and the colours blues, greens, soft reds, perhaps even some beautiful colours that you don't recognise... new colours, colours that belong to you, they are yours ... you feel the warmth of the sun, then a cooling breeze just touching your body... if you can sense it or imagine it, or hear your inner voice describe it, or just feel it, this means your secluded, safe place is there... and for you it is real ...

I want you to sense, see or hear that beautiful place. let it rest in your mind as if it were real, perhaps it feels like a memory, a memory of a past distant place that you know, a place that is safe, secure and comforting. A place where no one and nothing is able to disturb you, anything you want to imagine can be here, anything you don't want will have no power to manifest in this place... in this place is a pathway you know that as this pathway leads deeper into your garden there is more to learn, more to know... more to discover.

I'm going to count down from 10 to 1, I want you to imagine that you are moving down that path... going deeper into your garden as I count, with each and every number you hear, you feel your state of mental and physical relaxation doubling....going deeper and sounder becoming more and more relaxed with each count down.

Ten... just moving along the path, doubling that relaxation, moving toward that the inner part of your garden....

nine... going deeper now, all troubles and worries drain away, every time you breath out, you release a little more of the tension in your body and you relax more deeply and move down the path ...

eight even deeper now, going down, heavier and heavier... deeper and deeper As you move down the path, your body and mind follow you down, relaxing more with each number...

seven... go deeper now ...

Six... Deeper still ...

five.... Halfway down now ... doubling the relaxation with each count...

Every part of you deserves a deep rest, your conscious mind finally letting go of all worries, fears, apprehensions... all tension... just slips away into the air. Becoming nothing, melting into the aether... this is the time for your conscious mind to rest, to renew itself, doubling your relaxation at every step along the pathway... deeper now, more relaxed... so very relaxed now, you may even begin to feel a light, pleasant sensation in your hands or perhaps your feet... this is a sign that your blood pressure is settling down, that your blood is flowing smoothly throughout your body, a sign that the muscles are releasing small amounts of oxygen into your nervous system. the very fact that you can notice any feeling in your body is a conscious signal that it wants more of this, that it wants let go and double your relaxation again....

four...... deeper ... sounder , going down deeper still

three... as your body relaxes your mind has permission to relaxed as well... thoughts take a much needed rest.... your mind becomes quiet, you will still have thoughts, yet they will just pass through your mind, you'll notice them, acknowledge them, then just let them drift through, paying very little attention to them... and ... Notice now how much slower and more even your breathing has become...and as you notice that deep, quiet, breathing it is another signal for your mind to double to triple its relaxation....

two...Very relaxed now, doubling that relaxation again....mind, body, emotions all taking a much needed time out...

and one, Doubling your relaxation... very comfortable now, so peaceful, so wonderfully relaxed now...

during this time of deep relaxation, your subconscious mind can be aware of everything that is going on around you . . . any suggestions you hear will go directly into your subconscious mind, the suggestions that I give you, are for your benefit, in fact because we agreed on them before this session, we agreed on the direction they should take... they are accepted by the subconscious. . . These suggestions become locked in your mind . . . firmly fixed . . . deeply . . . in your inner mind . . . Implanted permanently, so these suggestions will remain with you . . . long after you open your eyes

. . . Helping you to change those things you want to change,. . . And these suggestions become new thoughts . . . helping you to change the things you want to change . . . And these changes allow you to enjoy your life . . . more . . . and . . . more . . . You are now becoming all that you are capable of being. You are able to let your creative side free, free of any fears or constraints that may have held it back, letting your subconscious tap into your super conscious and release the imaginative mind to physically manifest your latent abilities, ideas, dreams, fantasies and potentials so that you may fulfil your desires ...Your creative abilities are now being activated. Your latent creative abilities are beginning to emerge and intensify with each passing moment. You now draw upon all subconscious knowledge from your past to intensify you creative abilities... this may be from ideas you have had, secret thoughts you have entertained, movies you've seen, where certain scenes inspired you, books you may have read, or even things you have spoken about with friends... New fields of creative activity are now open to you... You are able to draw from unrestricted creative inspiration and energy... You now activate the creative ideas and thoughts ... You can now utilize your super conscious mind... You feel creative therefore you are creative...and here is the really amazing part, the beautiful part, you are in the process of creating a new individual. No matter what your age, no matter what your talents you can create, you can become, the exact person you want to become. You are everyday in every way becoming more and more creative.

You are creating a whole new positive individual. An individual who loves life, who feels good, who can evolve new ideas in the bedroom, new positions, new feelings and sensations ... You are creating a person who is mentally and emotionally not afraid to be creative, fun and enjoyable... the creation process never stops... you will not be the same tomorrow as you are today... you will not be the same today as you were yesterday. Nowhere is it written that you cannot change. You are able to change anything about your make-up any time you choose to... you can become those characters, take on those personalities you have always wanted, desired to be, wanted to be... Once you have decided what you want to be you will become that individual. you realize that what you think about is what the subconscious accepts, and you can recognize those traits within your own inner being... your subconscious accepts everything you put into it... you tell the subconscious exactly what you want and it will do exactly as you suggest...

Mentally repeat to yourself I want to become more creative, therefore I can mentally create a more imaginative person. I can be inventive, my imagination is fertile and always ready to try new things, my mind is abundant with new exciting ideas, it stimulates me and my imagination to come up with new ways of doing old things, new positions, new games new thoughts...

I will mentally create a powerfully creative person. I will allow myself to envisage new scenarios, if I what I can even take on new characteristics... become any character I want or have ever imagined... I am self-confident, my body and mind are active, I can become the person I choose to become because within me are all the traits that make it possible to know and believe that I will become what I think about.

In fact if you really think about it, the only reason you have found it difficult to be creative in the bedroom is because you haven't given yourself permission to be... we both know that you have the ideas, the desires the fantasies... you simply haven't allowed yourself to express them... so now you can, you can give yourself permission to be creative to have fun to reach out to your desires...

Once you do this you will realize that you are continuously developing, growing and becoming... and you also know that every thought ... and every suggestion given to your subconscious is acted upon. That every suggestion is real for you, that they have burned themselves deeply and permanently into your subconscious, where they will act upon the conscious mind, changing your thoughts, your habits and behaviours...

So now at the count of five you will return to full awareness, be wide awake feeling good feeling wonderfully refreshed and relaxed...

Continue to waking your subject up.

HYPNOTIC ORGASM OR THE HANDS FREE ORGASM

The following script combines many elements we have already discussed along with a few new techniques for you to learn as well. Before attempting this script make sure you are really comfortable with the process of hypnosis, that you know your subject really well even intimately. In the pre-talk stage ask you're subject to recall as vividly as they can, the most intense orgasm they have ever experienced.

Using anchors as we detailed earlier take them through stage by stage anchoring each part of the experience.

Let's assume you are going to anchor the earlobe (as this is a reasonably unique area a place not often touched) the subject recalls the experience at least twice. Now ask them where it was, where were you, as they describe the place, you will be eliciting as many details as possible while gently applying the anchor, a soft even pressure on the earlobe.

Can you remember the time of day or night, what smells were associated with the memory, where did it start in the body, were you nervous, were there any other people about?

With each answer from the subject squeeze the anchor point on the body.

Immediately after installing the last anchor reach up and gently close their eyes, gently push down and say ...

Close the eyes, Relaxing, deeply now...and look straight ahead, at the back of your eye lids as if it's a television screen. What do you see? ... (Let them describe what they see, even if it is nothing but blackness that's fine. Due to a thing called the hypnogogic effect a few people will see something) whatever they say just continue as it everything is normal *...that's correct, it is easy to focus your attention on the back of your eyelids, isn't it ... each second relaxes your body more deeply, more soundly ... and you already know how* *important it is to keep your eyes closed as you drift into a deep trance now. As you drift into a type of daydream state you may notice things beginning to appear on that screen at the back of your eyelids...but that's ok, you can just ignore them, let them drift or float, in, then out of your awareness...*

Now just take a deep breath, and relax... feeling the shoulders relax now... in fact the more you are aware of your breathing... the heavier those eyes become, heavier and heavier with each breath you take... I'm just wondering if you can visualize, that even though your eyelids are so relaxed and so heavy that they could be able to relax even more ... I wonder if in your imagination you could know what that feels like ... that the eyes could go ten ... twenty or even fifty times deeper, heavier ... down so soundly... so relaxed and sleepy now...heavier and heavier deeply soundly relaxed... those heavy, heavy eyelids... and staring at the deep darkness the greyness in front of you makes your deep relaxation and focus shift into trance... the more you focus... the deeper you go... and the deeper you go the more you are able to focus and block everything out except my voice ... the sound of my voice taking you even deeper, deeper and deeper down as you mentally make your eyelids even heavier, and heavier... until they completely lock down... closed, stuck tight, as if glued shut, held so tightly that no matter how hard you try to open them, they just stick even tighter, eyes so tightly closed ... in deep trance now.

Here you will notice one of two things, your subject will attempt to open their eyes, you see the eyebrows raise, as they test themselves. If this happens skip the next part. If they do not attempt any eye opening, say the following

Now, with your impossibly heavy eyelids ... closed so tightly and stuck so firmly, in a moment I want you to try to open your eyes, and find that they are stuck so completely that the more you try, the tighter stuck they become.

That's right. Keep trying to open them, and find that you cannot move your eyelids even the tiniest bit. They are frozen in place, no matter how hard you try to move them.

Try harder, now.

After a few seconds continue...

Very good.

You can stop trying now, and sink even deeper into trance now.

It feel so good to go deeper to become more and more relaxed... and you might have noticed the actual way the feeling of being so deeply relaxed, reminds you of how deeply hypnotized you are... and you might also notice that the awareness of being deeply relaxed sends you even deeper into trance... and so you can enjoy that pleasure even more now.

And now... that deeply relaxing stillness is spreading... from your eyelids, to your whole face. Your eyebrows, your nose, the muscles in the forehead and find that the muscles around your mouth are loosening, drooping, losing all tension. Your whole face is still... relaxed... heavy... feeling deep relaxation and comfortable.

And that pleasure, and that stillness ... and relaxation, spreads down, now... pouring down into your upper body, like a warm liquid, gently making its way down your arms, like thick, heavy, warm liquid... warm and relaxing and so, so smoothly flowing, deeper and with every passing moment, as if its filling the body like a vessel... you relax even deeper into your deep trance now

You might wonder which hand it will reach first... as it flows down into your upper body, arms, your elbows, your forearms, the wrists... warming and soothing them... as it flows it takes away all tension... you can feel it, warm and fluid, moving into your fingers.

You can feel moving into, filling your chest...it all across your stomach, and flowing down your hips.

At some point most people will experience some type of involuntary reaction, a finger twitch, a swallow, a body shift, you will use this to deepen the trance state

You might feel a last few little twitches in your fingers, now... before they relax completely, and grow completely still motionless deeply soundly relaxed.

You notice your body shifting its weight now, now... as it finally finds the most comfortable position to relax in and let go ... relaxing completely, and growing completely still motionless deeply soundly relaxed.

Whatever their reaction is incorporate it into your scripting

Now once again continue as normal

And now the heavy gel or thick liquid is flowing...further down through your body, moving into your legs... filling your thighs... your knees... and down your calves ...the shins. Pooling around your ankles, now, and pouring into your feet, between your toes. Filling your entire body now... with deep warm comfort, serenity ... calmness ...tranquillity, And you might take a moment to wiggle your toes a little, or flex or stretch your ankles, before the fluid settles, and your entire body, all of your body, is now completely relaxed....heavy...rigid......and still.

Excellent you are doing extremely well.

Now it's perfectly ok to just enjoy that deep, heavy, solid feeling... this deep, heavy, solid trance. Its ok to just take a moment and enjoy that feeling...When you think about trying to move... your body just becomes heavier... and that reminds you how very deeply hypnotized you are. Your deep trance now whenever you think about trying to move. It becomes even heavier, deeper, sounder, more solid and immovable.

There is a great sensation of comfort, deep pleasure even serenity filling your entire body and being right now...And as take a moment to enjoy that pleasure, as you live in that moment, you

will also notice that whenever you hear me say the word "deeper," all of those feelings increase, becoming stronger. It may take a moment for your body to relax completely, each time you hear me say the word "deeper". But will instantly begin looking forward to the pleasure of feeling your whole body quickly become warm ... and heavy... completely relaxed and tranquil ... And even deeper now.

Now to the reason you are here today, as you go deeper I want you to allow yourself to gently shift back in your memory, to a time when you had the most intense orgasm you can find in your memory ... take a moment to search for it... once you have that memory just remind yourself where you were, when it was...perhaps who you were with ... or if you can't remember an exact time imagine what your best most intense explosion of sexual release and energy would be like, who you would be with, what the situation would be, the time of day...

Focus on your body now, downward, Imagine the urgency centred in your clit, like an itch needing to be scratched but pleasurable... Now ... an urgency begins to build up in your body, images begin to flash through your mind, flashes of past experiences each has a feeling with it, of pressure and pleasure each flash is drawing you closer to that feeling of intensity it begins to build to get stronger ... an energy that is being drawn towards your crotch as you get closer to coming. You notice now that need ... urgency release ... where is it in your psychical body , is it everywhere, can you notice your heart rate increasing... between your legs, you know this feeling this sensation it that feels like nothing else on Earth, and it is as frustrating and it is delicious...

Now you begin to feel hot and cold at the same time. Erratic, irregular contractions begin in your muscles ... inside you...Your toes might curl, your breath shortens... your arms tense and you flex and contract muscles throughout your body, is this involuntary or an instinctive effort to bring on your orgasm.... Something your body just does when it gets ready to release... This is when you begin to make those little sounds, even if you don't mean to.

A sigh, then you have to draw in a gulp of air to get you're breathe back...then it comes again deep inside you...you feel a moan wanting to escape, perhaps it does escape... what do you do just a moment before you reach that final climax.... Does your body tense, do you make a sound, does your mind go blank or does it absorb itself in the sensation...what do you do right before you come, will it turn into a whimpering moan.

Now that intensity comes in waves rippling along the full length of your body tightening each muscle as it goes...first one then another following one after another, one...two...three.......four..............five, Then at last of all the energy that you've been drawing down to your clitoris and vagina arrives at the spot where you have been feeling the need ... it doesn't have a name, it just is what it is... and then you explode.

Something explodes in your brain, and your body at the same time... Your eyes roll back...you are panting trying to catch your breath but another wave of pleasure won't let you...you are frozen with intense pleasure, unable to move. The Legs stiffen, your back arches, and finally that moan escapes. The energy that you built up throughout the images, the smells, feelings even tastes... the memories are released all at once. Your inner muscles clench hard and rapidly, at the same pace as your elevated pulse. It feels incredible when that energy is released, like the pleasure you feel inside and between your legs when you're really aroused, multiplied a billion times. Have you had enough have you had too much? Yet there is still a part of you that wants more...

Your back arches again and your legs tighten almost to the point of cramping, and now it feels like your stomach is being sucked into itself... Now your inner muscles stop contracting ... your back relaxes, you catch your breath ... you feel as if you just had a very pleasant dream ... you're not quite awake yet. You're still floating ... in that peaceful state ... just below consciousness, ... and you're still holding on to the afterglow ... that tranquil euphoria ... your just letting your body enjoy the extra sensations as the intensity begins to fade .

When people say that the high they get from drugs is like sex, this is the part that they mean, those first ... few seconds after you've finished coming. And it's perfectly ok to enjoy those feelings...

In a moment, I'm going to count down from five to one. As I begin count, you will feel a tap! In the middle of your forehead, and that tap will break you out of the quietness you are experiencing right now, throughout your whole body. You will feel your body get lighter, more active, each count will bring you closer to full wakefulness. And at the count of one you will be able to move again, you will feel fully alert and wide awake, when you feel that tap in the middle of your forehead with each number that I count, you will wake up a little more from your trance, until at one you will be wide awake and feeling refreshed and alert.

Now. Continue as normal bringing your subject out of state.

ROBOT SCRIPT 2

In this script we will be incorporating the story telling concept. You don't have to use it, but I feel that it adds new wonderful elements to your hypnosis. The idea being to create a whole scenario not simply telling your subject they are a robot, by building in a back story the imagination of your subject comes into play.

After your induction...

And now you begin to become aware... even though your eyes remain closed, you begin to notice a slight awareness of your surroundings, cool air, perhaps you sense a wide open space, like a factory... in fact you become aware that you are in a factory, a large space... around you there is the slight hum of machinery, the movement of conveyor belts, you are on one of those conveyor belts... gently moving along, and now you notice there are no thoughts in your mind, simply an awareness of what's going on... but no actual thoughts... because you are waiting for thoughts ideas programming, you are waiting for software to enter you mind, to be placed there...

You are a robot, you have just been made, ready for the software , ready for the programming to be placed in your mind... to be placed in the circuits and functions that will become your mind. Telling you what and how to think, what and how to perform, act and behave... you are a robot... you have just been made... produced in the factory, ready to be programmed and then bought by an owner... n owner that has requested very special software to be inserted into your electro mechanical mind... you are a machine, designed to function as a machine, a robot you have no mind except your programming, no mind except your software... no thoughts except to obey that software, to follow your programming without a care or a thought, to simply follow orders and do as your software tells you...

That programming is being inserted now, as you move along the conveyor belt to a place where that software, that programming is inserted into your mechanical brain... no thoughts accept that which is programmed into you. No actions accept that which you're programming tells you to perform...

You feel a label being placed on your body, a code number, a bar code a production tag... confirming that you are a made product, produced to obey and serve, an automation, a product... a robot that has been made for a certain customer. A customer who has ordered a special robot a se machine, which means nothing to you... you don't care what you were made for, you have no feels or ideas about that matter, no thoughts, no thinking, no concerns because you ... just are ... you exist only to serve and obey... you are a robot. You are your programming, you are your software, and the tag proves it... so that whenever the tag is placed on you, it reminds you what you are... you are a product, a purchased machine, this is what the tag means ... the tag is proof of purchase a receipt for a product, a robot... an automaton, bought to serve and obey... whenever this tag is on your body that's what you are...a robot. A machine with not thoughts, just programming a series of functions designed to obey every command... a set of protocols ready to serve...

You now sense that boxing... packaging... movement, you are being transported along a service corridor to a loading bay... to your owner, the customer that has purchased you... you sense the gentle rumble of a truck, a delivery van, taking you to your new home... a new home where you will be the robot... performing the new operating system that is now in the place you will call your mind... your mind is not your own...your mind is software, programmed responses, obeying every command, that it is given, you arrive now, taken out of your box , packaging removed so that when you are switched on, you will open your eyes and be fully functional. Ready to obey, as you open your eyes and become functional you will take in your new surroundings, see your new owner and instantly your software will activate. You will as you open your eye become a fully functional automation, a robot, ready to obey and serve... at the count of three you will be activated... 1...2...3....

FREEZE

There is a bit of contention over many of the erotic hypnosis scripts, as long as you get your subjects agreement and permission all should be good. There is the theory applied by many hypnotists that all hypnosis is in effect actually self-hypnosis. Simply put, if you hypnotize someone telling them they will turn into a Mannequin, or freeze at your command. It may not work simply because they think: "No, I don't want to." Therefore communicate with your subject, as stated previously, make sure this is something they want. Talk it over, be attentive to the needs or kinky desires your subject.

According to the *All Hypnosis Is Self-Hypnosis Theory of Practise*, you are not commanding the subject, you can only act as a guide giving suggestions that they would agree to anyway.

This is of course only one theory, there is another that states, given the right suggestions with compliance from the subject you can make them do almost anything...

it's probably better to err somewhere in the middle, make your subject feel safe, make the idea exciting for them. This is assuming they haven't already asked to be turned into a mannequin. While it may be a turn on for you to have someone completely under your control, for many people, freezing, remaining motionless, or being a statue until someone releases undeniably has a certain anxiety or a feeling of helplessness.

After your induction

Just for a moment focus on you left arm... now imagine that your arm is a steel rod. See it feel it believe it... the arm is becoming stiffer more and more rigid, it is locking in position... Becoming frozen in space and time. The muscles becoming harder and harder, every sinew every fibre of the arm locking tightener and tighter. Solid, rigid, immovable. The arm is so locked so solidly frozen that it won't move, you can't move it... From now on, whenever I say the word 'Freeze to you' your body will become completely stationary, stuck, and immobile. That locked, solid immoveable sense you have in your arm now, will overtake your entire body ... You will not be able to move any part of your body, no matter how hard you try, it will be as though you have turned to ice, or solid steel, there is a force holding you in place. You will become a human statue, frozen ... locked... solid your body locked in position... a living statue.

You will be able to breathe normally, you will be able to feel everything that happens to you, and you will see everything that that is going on around you... yet you are a statue, a living statue you will be unable to turn your head, move a muscle, not even move a finger, you won't be able to utter a word... you will be unable to do anything... unable to do anything at all... whenever I say the word freeze to you, you will become a living statue...

Now focus on your right arm inside your right arm is an iron bar. See it feel it believe it... the arm is becoming stiffer more and more rigid, it is locking in position... Becoming frozen in space and time. The muscles becoming harder and harder, every sinew every fibre of the arm locking tightener and tighter. Solid, unbending, immovable. The arm is so locked so solidly frozen that it won't move, you can't move it...

Whenever you hear me say the word frozen it will be a trigger for you to freeze in place, to become a living sculpture Even though you are fully frozen ... You will be aware of everything that happens to you, and yet you will be completely trapped inside your body. I or Anyone else can move your body as they wish because you are a statue, frozen and stiff, unable to resist, locked in place, just simply a statue that others may move and position as they desire.

There is no choice, you won't be able to resist, no matter how you try, in fact you won't try, you are a statue, statues don't try,,, they just are ... no matter how you try or what you think about it, none of this will matter because you are trapped in your statue body, just staring out with the eyes, listening with your ears, feeling with your skin, but totally unable to move in any way. You will have no control whatsoever.

Now concentrate on your left leg notice it is becoming more and more rigid, solid .... See it feel it believe it... the leg indeed both legs now are becoming stiffer more and more rigid ... locking in position... each muscle becoming tighter Becoming frozen in space and time. The muscles becoming harder and harder, every sinew becoming tighter, every fibre of both legs locking tightener and tauter. Solid, inflexible, fixed immovable. Not to the point of cramping, they are simply following the rest of your body. Those legs locked so solidly frozen that they won't move, you can't move it...

Even though frozen your body still does the things it does automatically, breathing, blinking - all of those things will happen automatically. Even though your mind will be totally aware of everything that is happening to it, you will be completely unable to resist, as you are moved, in whatever way by whomever is around. They will be able to move you or place you however they want, like a mannequin in a store removing whatever clothes or putting on whatever they want.

Whenever I say the word 'Freeze to you' your body will become completely stationary, stuck, and immobile. You will become a living statue a living mannequin you will have no choice, no capacity to resist, no facility for movement at all ... until you hear the words "normal again (name of subject)", then and only then you will be able to move again, normally and freely, as if nothing had happened at all.

So right now your entire body is stiff, locked, frozen immovable just like it will be whenever you hear me say the keyword freeze.... See it your arms and legs locked in place, locked solid, only flexible when moved by somebody else ... feel the muscles of the back and chest lock into place, like cement ... only able to be moved by the will of others, a living posable mannequin... believe it... know it...

the entire body, from head to toe stiffer becoming more and more rigid, locking in position... Becoming frozen in space and time, each muscle becoming harder and harder, every tendon every fibre locking tauter. Solid, unbending, immovable. The entire body from head to toe is so locked so solidly frozen now that it won't move, you can't move it...

Whenever I say the word 'Freeze to you' your body will become completely stationary, stuck, and motionless. You will be fully aware of everything that happens to your body while it is frozen, while you are a human statue. Even though you have no control, your mind is still there, awake and aware, even while your body is totally and completely stationary even locked in place. This isn't a choice - you can't stop it or resist it. You will simply obey... Just as... you obey my voice now.

Whenever you hear me say FREEZE you will become a human figurine a mannequin, a statue like a statue you will have No choice, as a mannequin you will have no way to resist. Completely obedient and relaxed...watching through the eyes, experiencing everything yet with no ability to do anything. No choice, no way to resist. Completely obedient and relaxed...

For the moment just let the tension in your body ease off, just let all the muscles relax as you begin to return to normal... and as you relax, breathing deeply and normally allow the word FREEZE to become more and more deeply embedded in your subconscious, the suggestions I have given you here, today, are deeply embedded in your subconscious mind now, sealed in there like cement...permanent ... the word freeze is always there locked in your mind and always able to turn you into a living statue the instant you hear me say it, and leaving you that way until you are told to return to normal.

You can't stop it; you don't want to stop it. You have always enjoyed the idea... and you will continue to enjoy it, even looking *forward to the experience delighting in the exciting sensations of letting go, not having any control over your body, as a statue there are no responsibilities, no fears, no concerns you are just a thoughtless, mindless automation, a mannequin frozen in time and space, part of your enjoyment will come from this ... being unable to stop it... from having no choice, no free will, this is what will happen each and every time I use the trigger word freeze.*

You will become instantly and completely frozen, a human statue, to be altered, moved and used as desired. You will have no choice in this you will obey, always.

As your body relaxes fully now , returning to normal, each suggestion will stay deeply in your mind, there is no way to resist these suggestions, because they are what you really want, what you have always wanted, you have no choice but to obey and freeze when you hear the command. Your trigger word is now deeply, permanently locked in your mind so deeply, so permanently that you are completely unable to resist it.

You must obey. You will submit, the next time I use your trigger word you will freeze, trapped in your own body, completely unable to move on your own. And when they let you return to normal, you will remember everything that happened, having experienced it all. Having felt every hand on your body, every touch, every experience while you've been frozen in place.

But you have no choice while you are frozen. You will be totally frozen, unable to utter a word, unable to make any sounds at all.

You are a mannequin. A living statue, see it feel it believe it, Accept it. ... Yield to it now... This is your reality now...

Now wake your subject in the normal way...

PET

The idea of temporarily changing into an animal has been around for almost as long as humans have been gathering in places. Ancient shamans called it Shapeshifting, taking on the personality or features of an animal. Early Europeans had legends of werewolves or vampires transforming into bats. Even today the idea is a common feature of fantasy television shows. Popular books from Lost Boys to Harry Potter, feature all manner of shapeshifting. So if anyone ever tells you its weird... they are right ... but then it's also perfectly ok to be weird.

Animal roleplay or autozoophilia, is the act of imagining oneself to be an animal. The idea covers everything from kittens to pony play. It is not having relations with actual animals. That's something that books like this don't cover. If you are a Tibetan goat herder or Sherpa, performing the ritual of Dumje then by all means go for it, if you are not a Tibetan goat herder or Sherpa then you may need a type of therapy that is beyond the scope of this book.

As always talk to your subject find out what animal they want to identify with, as well as any other information they deem important, in short have them describe their fantasy to you. Then work this information into your script. In this example we are assuming your subject wants to be a kitten.

Another important consideration in animal roleplay is anchoring. It is important to add in the accruements of the animal being played, this adds another level to the erotic senses. Look at any pony play session and you will see leather harnesses, cats always have collars, cute ears or other little things that add to the realism or fantasy element. So wherever possible add these into your scripting. The script used here assumes that you have a small collar that is placed on your subject's ankle, a feeding bowl and a tail. You can use whatever anchors you like for your pet.

After you induction flow naturally into the script.

Imagine, for a moment, that you are no longer human. That you can be a kitten anytime you want or need to be. That you are a kitten. You might have the sensitive whiskers of a cat, or the playful attitude of the cat, or the curiosity. Just imagine what it would be like... just imagine what it is like...to be a kitten that's good, now for a moment imagine what would be needed to turn you into a cat, an adorable little kitten... a collar, well from now on wherever you wear this collar, on your ankle, not your other collar which wear on your neck for other reasons, but with this collar, you are a cat... the ankle collar has a little bell on it, you will hear it tinkle as you move, when you hear it you will feel even more feline, and cute and playful, you will feel even more like a pet an owned domesticated each time you hear the tinkle of the little bell on your ankle whenever it is on your ankle you will become a playful kitten, whenever you feel it on your ankle and know it's there ... you are a playful cat. As an obedient little kitten you will drink and eat from your pet bowl, each time you do you will feel more and more like a cat taking on all the traits and personality of a feline crawling on all fours, wearing your collar eating from your food bowl...and as a cat you will often be required to be naked, except for your collar and your ears or perhaps a tail. You will always be aware of your collar wearing the collar, hearing the bell... you will be happy to sleep at the foot of my bed or sleep in your pet bed or even being required to use a litter box, or go outside even being taken with other pets and owners to animal play events because as a pet and as an owned domesticated animal all these things are now your reality so whenever you wear this collar you will become a loving obedient pet...

Now at the count of five you will awaken ...

Continue to wake the subject as normal

EROTIC HYPNOSIS INDUCTIONS
THE SCRIPTS

Everything you have read up to this point has been to get you step by step closer to being able to perform these scripts confidently. You should by now have a fairly good idea of how and why these scripts work. The idea behind this section is that each of the scripts can be adapted to your particular needs or the needs of your partner/subject. For example a heroine script could be for any hero or heroine from wonder woman to black canary or in the case of a male partner batman, superman, whatever you like.

Each script is a guide to bigger better things, ideas or concepts limited only by your imagination.

Now that you are entering into the wonderful world of erotic hypnosis more fully there are a few things you will need to be aware of as you continue. I've said earlier that consent is tantamount to your success as a hypnotist. Therefore you will need the consent of anyone you hypnotise. Common sense and courtesy, you will also need to know what your subject wants from the session. Sit down have a long chat with them about their needs their fantasies or any desires they have.

Some people just want to get over basic fears, like anal, or doing it in public. Later you can deal with your own agendas or needs, wicked wishes or desires, but always start with what your subject wants or hopes to get from the experience. Not only is this polite it also helps to instil confidence and security in the subject, after all you are making it clear this is not all about you or your narcissistic needs... it's about them it's about what they want.

In fact to get what you want often requires helping the subject first for example using the stripper script is going to be a lot more effective if you have spent a session or two helping your subject feel good about themselves or have helped them loose weight or motivated them to go to the gym, a toned body looks better, feeling good fills your subject with enough confidence that there will be less hesitation or self-talk about not being a stripper, thus making the whole process easier.

OVER COMING PAST RELATIONSHIPS

As anyone who has ever been in a relationship will know, there is nothing more distracting or destructive to a current relationship than all the baggage bought from the last one. Or the one before that, or the one ten years ago that your partner still can let go of. The following script is similar to the previous one, I'm using it as an example of how you can adjust your scripts to accommodate different situations. It also serves to show how the Past Tense Principle or technique can apply to many situations. The example below also assumes that you have spent some time talking with your subject about what they feel when they think about the problem or what happens to them when they think about the past relationship. This is information that should be worked into your script.

Following immediately on from your induction

So just relax, letting go of the last of tension now…

You were telling me that for a long time you have been experiencing a problem which you have found difficult to control, and that problem was (name the specific person, alternatively state the year, or other detail that you and the client both will know as representing the past relationship.)

Then you decided to use your own mind your powerful subconscious mind, gaining control over this. Because it was in fact your subconscious mind that caused you to have all those negative thoughts and reactions. And then having made the decision to gain control over it you did…

You already know that your conscious mind is in control of all your thoughts, while your subconscious mind governs the autonomic nervous system. It regulates your breathing and your heartbeat and your tension … when you're tense the flow of blood to your muscles increases, making you more tense, then that tension causes more blood to flow to your muscles, and around the cycle goes…

So let's go back a step...let's take a moment to look at what you were thinking about, in the conscious mind that caused your subconscious to react the way it did. What were you thinking about, what did you just allow into your mind, what are the thoughts that triggered your body to react...

And as you think about this, take a moment to examine whether it was images, or feelings that started it... did memories come in flashes, pictures, images, did your body tighten up, did your breathing change, when you allowed those images to enter your mind... did the body become tense... when that memory came to mind did your muscles tighten... in the past did you allow your memories to control you...

Even though you know that's all they are, just memories, and memories can't physically harm you in any way... just memories, memories can't actually harm you in any way...they are as easy to let go of as any type of discomfort... you can easily and simply let them go... and now you have, these memories used to bother you once, a while ago, but then you made the decision to let them go and you did... you chose not to be hurt by them anymore and you weren't hurt or effected by them anymore...

Now wake the subject as per normal

The last few paragraphs of this script are the most important. You are actually stating two things at the same time. Both are important. Firstly you are speaking in past tense, while creating a subtle form of dual reality. ***Did your body tense when you thought of this?*** Which is another way of saying "so you used to tense up a bit, but you're not doing that now right!"

THE SCRIPTS EXTRA BITS

This section assumes that you are now a confident hypnotist. That the process is familiar to you that you do not need constant explanations of each and every detail of how or why a script works. This section will not feature whole scripts but parts or hypnotic phrasing that you can employ or inject into your existing ideas and scripts to make them better and more effective. Some of them are just fun fantasies or to spark your own ideas. Although you will find some of them are advanced they should only be used if you know your subject well and have prior agreement with them that what transpires is OK with them. You will have built rapport with a lot of trust before adding these extra lines to your work as an erotic hypnotist

LINES THAT CAN BE ADDED INTO YOUR SLAVE HYPNOSIS SESSIONS

You can think of nothing but pleasing your master. You want nothing else ... your only desire is to please him. You desperately want to please him, to do anything for him. You love serving him, you love being available to him you want it completely... you need it... in some ways it's like breathing, you cannot live without it... You know all this is true. Whenever you think of sex, you will think of being a slave, you will open up top your true self... you will visualise and imagine being used... of being owned... of serving and you will think of even feel the pleasure you will get from this you will feel your love of it overpowering your feelings. Whenever you think of it, you will feel intense joy. Always when you think of it, you will feel happy and thankful that you belong to your master.

So just let your eyes close now.... don't even think about it, just let them close all by themselves as if that's what they wanted to do... let my voice guide you easily and smoothly ... gently... caressingly... into a state of submission.... don't even think about that either, just allow it to

occur as if it has always been what your mind really wants...submission to unrestrained pleasure.... pleasure you have always wanted....

You become aware of your inner most mind now... you can choose to continue in that dreamy state and enjoy that feeling... the feeling of being someone else.... the feeling of letting go, letting go and releasing that fantasy you have always dreamed about, the who and what you have always wanted to be ... of being different.... of being free to enjoy your most intimate fantasies.... to become real for you....

You will always be able to hear the words that I use, then as your mind becomes absorbed in those images you've created... perhaps you will find that you don't focus so much on the words that I use, but only those words that your subconscious needs to hear. What does your subconscious need right now, does it need to let go of the day to day struggles and worries... does your subconscious need to open itself up to your true desires and needs? There is a part of you that already admits, perhaps quietly to yourself, that you are a slave

This will make you VERY excited. There is nothing more exciting for a woman than to be completely under the control of the man she loves, there is nothing more arousing than to have completely surrendered to him. This is true isn't it

And you now know you are deep in trance, there is no uncertainty about it at all. You are in a deep, profoundly deep trance ...In fact, you now understand that you are completely and perfectly under my absolute control. In fact you are now just a passenger I am driving! From this point you conscious and subconscious mind are being driven by my words and my words only. Whatever I say to you is your reality. It is totally and completely real for you. For the time of this session and any future sessions when we are together.

You can think of nothing but pleasing your master. You want nothing else only to please him. You desperately want to please him, to do anything for him. You love serving him ... being this way with him, serving him is all that matters. You love being good for your master. You love it completely. You know all this is true. Whatever you think of sex, you will think of your master... whenever you think of being submissive, you will think of him, whenever you think of being used, you will think of him ... you will feel your love of him because he enables you to be who you really are...and who you really are is a slave, property, knowing this will overwhelming your emotions. Whenever you think of it, you will feel intense happiness comfort and peace because you have really finally found your place. Anytime you think of it, no matter where you are or what you're doing ... you will feel happy and thankful that you belong to him.

You probably are finding it a little more difficult to think right now. This is normal. Your subconscious mind is now imprinted with your service to your new Master. Any and all thinking both subconscious and conscious locks your body and mind upon a new destiny. You are to become a slave, a slave to my wishes and little more than an empty headed slave. Property and object of desire

LINES THAT CAN BE ADDED INTO YOUR BDSM HYPNOSIS SESSIONS

A personal fantasy session involving a kidnapping fantasy

And now as if in a half dream...you can allow your imagination to run free... you find yourself in a large room... somewhere... somewhere you have never been before.... the room is dim... quiet.... you sense something strange has happened.... you become aware of people near you.... people moving quietly.... -someone comes close.... you can feel the heat of their body.... they are leaning across you... you suddenly realise your arms are being held above your head... you feel rough cloth scratch across you skin.... you are naked... leather straps are being tightening around your wrists... faceless hooded figures seize your ankles and you feel the straps tightening... you are bound... helpless... naked...

LINES THAT CAN BE ADDED INTO YOUR INDUCTIONS

Just Forget about any distractions. Just let them slip through your awareness, notice them then let them pass through without a second thought... Let go of any unwillingness to experience this completely. Trust me ... and have confidence in yourself so this will work. You can clear everything else from your mind... and allow the hypnosis to happen ... all you have to do is focus on my voice... let it take you down deeper and deeper ... Imagine for a while that the rest of the world does not exist, that it does not matter just for the time you have allowed yourself to go into deep trance... all other thoughts drift away, they may distract you for the briefest moment but then you realise they are not important now. Forget everything else that is going on, outside noises sounds, thoughts, concerns or worries... all you need to be concerned with are my words, knowing that they will take you as deep as you want to go... all other thoughts drift away far, far away, Nothing matters but how deeply, soundly you can enter trance now.... Your only thought is how deeply you can enter a state of trance now...

The above is another good example of a CHC **enter trance now** is both a suggestion and a command

Focus on your breathing, breathe deeply and slowly, in and out, in and out. Relax and keep going, in and out, in and out. Let your body relax, let the tension slip away from your muscles.

As you relax, you will no doubt hear outside noises or distractions...if you hear anything... that distracts your mind from focusing and relaxing...you will find that you can easily use that noise as a cue to bring your thoughts and your awareness back to the place of peace and tranquillity that you experiencing right now.

Just allow that feeling of relaxation to spread.... all the way through your body... you are doing extremely well now... and your body will respond at exactly the right speed for you... everything you are feeling now is the way it should be...

LINES THAT CAN BE ADDED INTO SEXUAL ENHANCEMENT SESSIONS

You are going on a journey... this is not an imaginary journey... this is a journey into something you already are... and have always been... a journey deeper into who you really are, the time of denying your true self...your true desires has past... you are going into the full experience of sensual pleasure.... you are going to enjoy being a woman.... you are going to allow yourself to be...fully and completely a woman, a creature of sexual pleasure and energy you are from this point on going to stop denying the secret pleasures of a woman's body... you are now no longer trapped by feelings of guilt or social constraints or expectations of other people...you are going to fully accept the experiences and all the feminine sensations you have imagined and dreamt of... there are no boundaries.... no limits... you are entering a state where you are free to be what you want to be... to feel what you want to feel...

I want you to imagine taking in the fragrance of the opposite sex, perhaps it is an alluring perfume or aftershave. Possibly it is a clean freshly washed smell. Perhaps it is the stimulating smell of sex as it travels so easily to your nose ... Allow the aroma to simulate you... to excite you. It happens so easily, that you feel yourself getting excited by the idea that you can be aroused in such a way. In fact, as the scent increases now, you find your arousal level grows with each word you read and find it easier and easier to just follow my words and enjoy the sensations I give you now. You are not even wondering about anything, but the erotic aroma around you now. It is like a wonderful exciting alluring hand guiding you and making you even more turned on now. You are now ready for the next test.

Imagine a woman/man standing in front of you, the most erotic woman/man you have ever seen. This can be any erotic person you can imagine or have imagined s/he could be a film star. They might even be a porn star... this could even be a friend. Someone, anyone you have secretly thought about, there is no need for anyone but you to know who this person is... you can keep their name and image locked in your mind for no one else to see except you... but right now this person talking to you...they are saying very sexually stimulating things they know exactly what to say to you to get you thinking, to get you excited at the possibilities of what may happen.... You are very excited by their voice, their words, they know exactly what words to use...and how to say them... and now you give yourself permission to be excited by this. You give yourself permission to be erotic with this person. And even though this is pure fantasy you know that it feels good to feel good you are allowed to feel good and it feels good to feel this way...

You already know that each climax you have will lead you to another each climax feeding into the following powerful orgasm, every time you cum you will want to cum more ... You want to come again and Again riding that powerful wave of pleasure for as long as you can.

You want to come, you want to beg for it. You will find that the words slip from your lips unconsciously please let me come master, master Please let me come. And even though you feel as if you cannot wait for permission. You must wait for permission. You must always wait for permission to orgasm...and only when I give you permission are you able to cum...

A FEW FINAL NOTES

THE MASTER INDUCTION

What I' am about to share with you may at first seem a little out there, even unbelievable it does however work and it works rather effectively. It is the pinnacle of all you're learning as a hypnotherapist/hypnotist if you apply the following induction as close to word for word as you can, with confidence, surety it will place about 99 percent of people into the trance state in under 30 seconds.

It may take years to get his right to perform it well, because basically it is performance. You will have seen stage hypnotists do this and it kind of spooky to watch, it involves all the principles we have discussed in this book and a few others that should become obvious once you do it.

The only real trick is be confident be so convicted within yourself that this will work that there is no doubt in your mind. Any doubt will translate over to your subject and make it difficult.

It is also one of those things that is very hard to describe. Like the force in star wars you can't really teach it, you have to experience it ... by doing it. No I'm not saying it's the force. Although it can look like that, it is an effect based on the dual reality principle used in mentalism and stage hypnosis.

The effect will hypnotise anyone, anywhere if you play it right. Once again we assume that you have been asked to demonstrate your incredibly amazing powers as a hypnotist. A volunteer is selected, you separate your volunteer from the main group of people (spectators) far enough away that they can still see what's going on, yet cannot hear what you are saying to your subject.

Now have the subject stand up straight, lean in and whisper to them,

Ok you're going to get hypnotised, is that ok your good with that right? You're getting permission here. *All you need to do is*

follow my instructions to the letter, do exactly as I say and you will go into trance and I promise you'll really enjoy the experience. As your taking place your hand just behind them on the nape of their neck, the idea being that you are going to tilt their head forward on cue.

Ok good now close your eyes and rest your head... as you say this tilt their head forward so that it drops, *and do exactly as I say, just relax your shoulders now your chest... let your arms become heavy and even though you remain standing go deeper now...*

That's It.! You have just learned one of the most powerful; and amazing demonstrations of hypnosis. It works due to the dual reality principle, the spectators are far enough away that they cannot hear exactly what you're saying to your subject, they may pick up small parts of it, yet not hear all of it. What they see is you talking to the subject when suddenly their head tilts forward he or she is seen to relax deeply and fall into trance. While your subject is simply following your instructions. The dual reality is the audience seeing one thing and believing it while your subject is believing another thing altogether.

The next step is as you keep talking to your subject

t you begin a normal induction until they willingly fall into a real trance through the compliance principle.

STRANGE PLACES, STRANGE DEEDS

Imagine the weirdest place you can have sex... or the naughtiest thing you could once in that strange place.

For some this can be as extreme as doing it in a glass elevator while thousands of unsuspecting shoppers look on, for others it will be pouring orange juice, custard or some other squishy food over each other's bodies then licking it off.

The key factor many people miss is timing, it's not so much the where, as the when, when is the right time to do these crazy things. In the case of the master or dominant, the right time is when I say it is... therefore this script instils an instant state of high sexual arousal in your subject. A state that with a few sessions becomes so extreme, so intense that the subject will want to do it anywhere any time.

Posthypnotic suggestions might include

Whenever I pull your hair you will instantly submit, get wet, turned on you will be ready to obey me

COVERT HYPNOTIC LANGUAGE PATTERNS FOR EVERYDAY USE

Contrary to popular opinion it is possible to make people think in a certain way, to feel good about helping you, joining you in your quest or even putting effort into projects that they might not even have considered under normal circumstances.

Cult leaders do it, the thing we remember most about Hitler and other charismatic political leaders, was their seeming supernatural ability to excite and inspire individuals even an entire nation.

Successful public speakers and motivators are able to develop these mysterious skills as a trait, advertising companies have mastered the art of making us feel or believe things, even take certain actions, sometimes over and above common sense.

This section of the book will show you some of the most advanced techniques for getting people to agree with you, to think that your ideas are good, in fact done correctly some people will even think that your ideas are better than average. These methods can also be adapted for getting people into trance state easily and quickly

While none of these techniques are particularly hard or difficult to learn very few people are aware of them, each of us may know one or two that we use almost randomly or accidently as we travel through life, using them ad hock, putting them down to coincidence. Perhaps you figured that if you could get people to smile they were more inclined to agree with you or to go along with your way of thinking. On the negative side many people discover early in life that various types of emotional blackmail get things to go their way. The problem being that even though these people may get what they want, it is temporary, leaving people eventually feeling bad about helping them.

Some of these techniques are so simple, so easy to apply that you will probably wonder why you didn't think of them yourself, others will take some explaining, the psychology or understanding of human behaviour that creates them or makes them so effective.

They will all take practice along with a readjustment of how you have been communicating and thinking.

There is no guarantee that these patterns will work one hundred percent of the time, you must take each situation as it comes, mixing and matching, working on every aspect of your communication from timing the technique, to the tone you deliver them in, to the order or choice of words you use.

As a stage hypnotist I started using these techniques in my show I found that many people would become hypnotized to various levels *before* being invited on stage to be part of the show.

Actually on many occasions people in the audience would fall under during the middle of the show. Other hypnotists began asking me what I was doing.

About the same time I had several therapy clients who for various reasons needed better communication skills, more effective ways of getting their point across or developing relationships. Some of these clients were business people others were individuals or couples, I started teaching privately almost in secret how to apply these techniques, the results for those clients where astounding, others, usually my corporate sales or hypnotherapist friends and one acquaintance who was simply a manipulating son of a ... suggested strongly that I not include this section in the book. The fear being that I would be giving away far too many secrets. Ill express to you, the reader the phrase that I told each of them.

With Great Power Comes Great Responsibility

We communicate on many levels, whether we realize it or not, words affect us emotionally.

Interpersonal communication is where we talk to ourselves, intrapersonal communication is where we talk to others either individually or in groups. The words we use in both these situations can change the entire feel and meaning of our message.

When we chat away to ourselves we are often talking ourselves out of really good ideas, as a hypnotherapist and counsellor I have helped many clients and friends readjust their internal dialogue.

Getting those people to be more positive, make better life choices and create action in their lives. Simply by changing the way they speak to themselves.

As part of the process and so that they fully understood what I was talking about I would give small examples, examples of how words effect emotions and how a simple sentence can deeply affect us. These small examples proved so effective and fascinating that people kept asking for more.

On stage as both a hypnotist who does charity shows and as a mentalist my job is to screw with people's minds. From making you think a certain thing on cue to reading what you are most likely thinking. Once again not only is this fun for the audience and for me as an entertainer but people keep asking me how I do what I do.

This book is the first step in the culmination of some thirty plus years, not only of research but actually applying these techniques and helping others apply them... Some of these techniques may appear hypnotic, almost magical in their effectiveness others will take many hours of practice.

Using them properly and adapting them to your life, communicating style and needs will not only be fun, it will increase your possibilities make you a better communicator and give you an advantage in most situations

Are these all my ideas?

No, we all stand on the shoulders of those that came before us... these techniques are not new, much of this work is based on the work of many incredibly gifted fore runners in NLP communications hypnotherapy and other fields such as psychology. Luminaries such as Robert Dilts, Richard Bandler and of course Milton Erickson, all I did was apply them, use them and later adapt and create my own techniques something you to will be able to do as you practice them,

How to use this book and the techniques

You can read the whole book through once, or the recommended several times, to get a handle on the techniques then choose one or two techniques and get out there and practice, practice, practice.

Where ever possible I will explain the psychology behind a technique, what the effect on the mind and emotions is. Along with different examples of how they might be used in business, personal relationship even in some case its therapeutic use, perhaps even how I utilize these techniques on stage during a performance. Because the more you understand the easier it will be to apply them

Thus giving you enough information to adapt each to your specific needs

THE SOUP

As you work through these ideas and concepts you will discover that many techniques are not designed to be used alone. You can mix and match them as you go, a simple ten minute conversation can involve numerous applications all working together to make somebody feel or behave differently

KNOW YOUR OUTCOME

You must know what it is that you want achieve, when applying any of these techniques. Have a goal in mind and work toward it. Many people already know a smattering of these techniques and we all know a salesman who uses them. Most of us however stumble through conversations not really knowing what to say next, let alone what the result might be. This is one reason why so many men are shocked or caught off guard when their wives or partners have issues. And want to "talk"

DELIVERY

We communicate on five main channels

VOICE

BODY LANGUAGE

TONE

TIMING OR PACE OF WORDS

CHOICE OF WORDS

Many of these techniques will employ more than one of these principles or channels, this is where practice comes in, developing your own pace and style of speaking or using the skills as you learn them. Don't expect to get it right straight away, work at it, be willing to adapt and not get stuck in one way of doing things

As you apply these techniques you are going to have a direct effect on a person's state of being, mostly you will affect whether they feel...

Good or bad about something

**Their self-image
What they believe
Their memory
What they do next
In some cases the actual functioning of the brain**

Plus a whole lot more

Rather than detail all these now and the process of soup I will now get to the techniques, explaining as we progress through the book. Remember practice them, enjoy them, many of them will be directed at you and how you can communicate more effectively with your inner self. Only use them for good, creating positive change in a person has more rewards, getting them to do more for you than any other method. If you can bring a smile to one person each day and help to improve their life you will be doing what we call creating memories

Keep in mind that at the end of time, all you or anybody else will be is, a memory, that's all you can leave behind, those memories are far more powerful and meaningful than any riches you may be fortunate enough to leave as a legacy. So therefore if you are actually going through life creating those memories, then why not create the very best ones.

I WAS WONDERING TECHNIQUE

Let's start with the basics; this technique is a good place to begin the technique gives you power in any conversational situation because it removes the pressure from the speaker and the listener.

We can soften any negative statement by applying it. Hide a direct command in a sentence that starts with it (we call this front tagging) and it provides you with an escape clause when speaking your mind and find that the other party starts disagreeing with you.

Keep in mind that the first rule of any communication process is not what you say; it's what the other person hears. What is heard determines the nature of your message.

For example in my clinical work I might ask or state to a client that

'I was wondering if you are ready to give up smoking today',
Or
'I was wondering if you will give up smoking today'.

At this stage two very important things have occurred firstly I've issued a CHC or hidden command it's designed as a normal statement.

"Give up smoking today"

Secondly I haven't issued it as a command because as far as the listener is concerned 'I was just wondering'.

This technique can be used when asking a husband to mow the lawn or a wife to clean the house (not that you don't) these are just examples

I was just wondering if you will mow the lawn today

Or we can soften the statement by saying

I was just wondering if you will be able to mow the lawn today

As we learn more of these techniques we are going to use our soup and combine or mix many techniques showing you how to deliver this more effectively

Another example I use in my clinical hypnotherapy work is as a client enters the office I might state

I was wondering if you are finding it easier to relax now

Again I will not use this technique by itself I will soup it combining it with my knowledge of the client mixing it with several other techniques. This is done is a natural conversational way that is comfortable and relaxing for the client and makes my job a lot easier.

We will return to these examples throughout the book showing you how to adapt them creating a language soup that truly affects peoples

In the dating situation you might use the phrase *"I was just wondering what you were doing next Friday"* or *"I was just wondering what you are drinking"*

Placing a tag at the beginning of a statement changes it into something else entirely. Next time you are in a heated debate with a loved one (as it is with our loved ones that most heated debates occur) instead of reacting to your emotions and scream

"Listen here you misdiagnosed piece of renal crap shut up so I can speak"

Instead say something to the effect of,

I was just wondering if there is a better way we can handle this

Another example from therapy is how many weight lose clinics will apply this simple front tag to motivating their clients.

Rather than saying

Ok let's lose some weight

Many are now asking

I was wondering what the best way for you to get to your ideal weight might be?

This works on many levels it appeals to the inner nature of the client and gets them involved they become part of the process; it also reframes the situation it is now not about losing extra weight it is now about gaining an ideal weight.

This is a reframe or a reversal and by the end of this book you are going to fall in love with them, they are one of the most powerful techniques for altering what you are saying into something that is heard

Finally there are right and wrong ways to use this technique it will take a little practice and you must feel or read each situation as it occurs, for example in the dating situation it might not be correct to say ***"I was wondering if I could buy you a drink"*** as you will learn as we progress through the techniques this statement is closed and may result in a negative response such as

"No you can't buy me a drink"

Whereas asking

'I was wondering what you are drinking'

Implies an answer of either coke or the preferred alcoholic beverage, you may be asking for a completely different reason.

Similarly while

"I was wondering if you would go out with me on Friday"

Is more powerful than

"Will you go out with me on Friday?"

It can still get a negative response as opposed to

"I was wondering what you are doing on Friday"

This should cause the listener to respond with, whatever it is they have planned for Friday night or a statement that alerts you to the fact that they may be available on Friday such as

"I really don't know I have nothing planned"

The point of this short and direct lesson is to alert you to the fast that, placing certain tags at the front of your statements will alter the feel of and reaction to the statement, as you move through these pages you will discover many more

SHUT UP

There is nothing worse than being labelled as a manipulator, even if you were trying to manipulate someone into doing the right thing, the word manipulation has a bad rap people don't like to feel that they were cohered into action either positive or negative, this first technique offers you an "out" in the early days of applying these techniques and because more and more people are becoming aware of them you may find the occasional person accusing you of using some sort of mystical influence, here you can always answer with "no not at all I was just wondering that's all"

In the erotic induction process you might use the statement

"I was just wondering if you can recall your strongest most powerful orgasm"

"I was just wondering if you can learn to let go of those inhibitions that were holding you back"

I was just wondering what it feels like to let go"

Each of these and others we will discuss can be gentle worked into both the testing or convincing stages and the induction.

THE 'MAYBE' TECHNIQUE

As described in the I was wondering technique, the maybe technique provides you with an "out" in this case you're not making a statement that could be argued with you are asking a question that requires some type of answer.

Maybe you will learn to use these techniques. Maybe you will combine these first two techniques into applications that will help you to communicate more effectively

Maybe you'll clean your room today

In the therapy situation I might use statements like

Maybe you'll learn to relax today

Maybe you'll learn to listen to your wife more

Maybe you'll be able to be more relaxed around this issue with your husband

And the classic

'Maybe you'll dream up new ways of being successful tonight'

The maybe technique is an internalizing technique; it is very difficult for a person to hear such a statement without looking inside themselves and wondering whether or not the statement may be true.

Naturally there are different levels of this, some statements might not be right for everyone, the better you know a person the more likely you are to adapt your speech and create sentences that affect them.

YOU PROBABLY ALREADY KNOW THIS

You probably already know how effective these techniques are and you are probably already thinking of ways to use them in your daily life

Now that you have a few "outs" and have seen how they can affect a person's state or mind set, it's time to practice a statement that actually causes a change in what the person is thinking or feeling.

Like any good hypnotherapist I have a really comfortable chair in my office

During therapy sessions as a client sits in the chair I will say something like

You probably already know how comfortable these chairs are

Or during my stage show s volunteers are coming on stage for the induction I will casually state

You probably already know that great shows involve many volunteers

Or

You probably already know that you're going to get up on stage tonight and be the star of the show...

You probably already know how easy it is to relax and let go of your tension

And later

You probably already know how good it feels to relax

Such statements are delivered so casually they bypass the normal restrictions of the conscious mind and the volunteers actually feel that yes they do know at some level just how nice it feels to relax. Those who just casually thought about getting up on stage now believe or feel that they were thinking about it all night.

Parents can use this effectively to get kids to clean their rooms

You probably already know how much better it is to have a clean and organized room, how much more fun it is,

In relationship counselling I might turn to the husband and say

You probably already know how much easier it is to listen to your wife and let her get things off her chest, deal with her feelings and just air things,

what happened here is that the important statement has been hidden in a larger statement this helps it to bypass the conscious reasoning and sneak in, the husband will believe that he does know this even if he has never actually had the experience,

A good example of how effective this can be is the wheelchair incidents. Over the years I've had many clients who are restricted to wheel chairs for various reasons. (Notice I said restricted to, we will look a reframing a bit later on)

Several felt that because they were in this situation they had trouble meeting members of the opposite sex, actually meeting and chatting weren't the problem it was developing a relationship. Thus the following sentence was constructed for them

You probably already know how much fun a wheel chair can be

One client even used it to pick up girls, he would begin normal light hearted chatting then once it developed to the stage where he was going to ask for a date, yet felt that for various reasons the lady in question would start coming up with excuses, he would actually say that sentence

You probably already know how much fun a wheel chair can be

And resistance to him and he's chair dropped Steve ended up getting a lot more dates began feeling better about himself and eventually married

Now is a good time to mention softening. As a mother you might feel inclined to use this technique on your children by stating

'You probably already know that if you don't clean your room your father is going to flail the skin from your body and sell you into slavery.'

As a therapist using these techniques one might be inclined to say

'You probably already know that you are going to die a horrible painful death if you don't stop smoking'

Or

'You probably already know that if you don't listen to your wife she is going to have an affair with the guy who cleans the pool'.

Or

'You probably already know that being restricted to a wheelchair is not the end of the world'.

You get the idea, these are all negative statements, and even if they are meant to be positive they will come across as negative and have a result that is totally opposite to what you wanted

Think about what you're saying construct each phrasing carefully, know what it is you want to achieve, know your outcome

'You probably already know how much easier you will breathe and take in air once you give up smoking'

'You probably already know how much more pleasant things are when you listen to your wife's needs'

'You no doubt already know how much better you'll feel when you get to your ideal weight'

I'll give you an example of just how powerful this technique can be in therapy I had a client many years ago who had a problem with drinking, he considered himself an alcoholic and had tried various STEP programs to no avail.

It turns out he wanted to stop drinking, yet not give up other parts of his life. Most of these programs involved giving up virtually everything connected to the drinking.

After talking for an hour or so I constructed a sentence, simply one line, a virtual throw away statement that rewired his brain on so many levels that he was able to rethink and start the process of taking control of his drinking

He took personal authority over his habits and reported to me later that he had perhaps never actually been an alcoholic, he just needed to be more aware of himself his own limitations and have more control in his life, and the sentence was this

"Well Peter, you probably already know, what it feels like when your body is sending you signals, that it's had enough to drink and it's time to stop".

From this point on Peter found it easy to listen for those signals he became aware of them, they had always been there Steve simply hadn't been aware of them or had chosen not to listen to them.

Delivered at just the right time in the conversation, in just the right way this simple sentence managed to have a positive effect on the rest of Steve's sessions with me and his life. As a therapist *you probably already know when the best time to deliver these statements is, don't you*

What the 'you already know' statement does is, it changes the minds inherent need to reject information that it doesn't feel good about, causing the listener to look inside and check whether or not they do already know this, this mental act of looking inside may only last a second or two but it has the effect of tuning into the sensations coming from the body and connecting them to the statement just heard.

We can tag doubtful or unsure statements with this technique making them project into the mind of the listener more effectively

You can trust me

I won't cheat on you

My plans for this business will work

Time will heal this

Are all statements that if delivered straight might cause the listener to feel worried or concerned about something, even if they are unsure exactly what those worries are.

Now listen to them again with the you already know tag

You probably already know from experience that I won't cheat on you

You probably already know that my plans for this business will work

You already know that you can trust me

You know that time will heal this

Even just by reading these lines you can almost feel the different in the approach and delivery of each of these statements, the tag turns things that are unsure in nature into believable statements even when they might not be one hundred per cent accurate they will feel as if they are.

We all love to hate complements

Here's a simple experiment you can do at home,

Next time your partner comes out all dressed up from twelve hours of getting ready and putting on her makeup, if she is female or if he is male a five minute cloths throw session.

Change your compliments using the tags we have learned instead of saying

You look really nice today

Say something like

You know what that outfit does for me

It's a reframe or reversal of the complement, normally if you say you look nice you will get a response like

OHHH this old thing

Or I can never feel good about how I look

Reframing it with this tag still delivers the complement yet now there is no arguing, it's about what the dress does for you not how it makes them feel and look it's about how it look to you and makes you feel.

She will spend the rest of the night feeling that she has had a complement and feeling good about herself.

I've had occasion to train sales people in many of the techniques used in this book, many have successfully adapted the statement tag for example

You probably already know how this computer will increase your effectiveness at work.

Or

You probably already know how much better games look with this graphics card

Let's assume that your partner is suspicious that you may be cheating or be spending too much time checking out the opposition and to reassure them you say

"You have nothing to worry about"

Chances are they will immediately think that they do have something to worry about

As opposed to the statement

You know you have nothing to worry about

This simple tag at the front of the statement can change the whole feeling of that statement we can make it even more powerful by reversing it

You know it makes me feel more secure in us, when you worry like that

This what we call an 'ambiguous statement' or phrase it can mean many things on many levels we will talk about them more later, for the moment though, unless you stupidly deliver it in a tone of sarcasm, it will rewrite your partners internal feelings about the whole situation, it effectively redirects the concerns away from you having a roving eyes to how it makes her feel.

Just as a personal note; if you are checking out other women with the intention of finding a new partner don't waste your time or your present partners, do both of you a favour, move on

Another therapeutic situation might be weight loss, where statements like

You probably already know how much healthier you feel when you are your ideal weight

Is very powerful creating a mindset that leads to the client being happier about making choices that will result in weight loss,

In the dating scene

This is a brilliant technique practice have fun with it, always lean toward the positive in what you're saying and you probably already know that this will work for you

On a deep level you probably already know how effective these techniques can be, here you are adding a definite command to look inside to examine your feelings about whatever is being said as you.

Using the technique you will soon develop your own style of pacing and delivering them, even perhaps to the point where it becomes natural for you to speak and construct your sentences or statements of intent in new ways, on a deep level you already knew this didn't you.

The part of the statement that works is the

'On a deep level' tag at the front

This directs the listener to things that are already known and even if the statement might not be strictly 100% true it will be connected to something that is true for the listener.

DON'T TOO QUICKLY TECHNIQUE.

Telling someone not to do something usually has the opposite result, tell a teenage male to be careful and he will most likely start taking stupid risks. This information about basic human nature can be used to great advantage in hypnotic practise. Telling them not to rush or to slow down will more often than not make them speed up the process.

Don't relax too quickly
Don't submit too quickly
Just take your time
NEGATIVE WORDS
Over the years that I've been practicing therapy with people, I've taught many of them how to readjust their internal dialogue, it seems

that we are constantly talking ourselves out of what are really good ideas, like starting a business going back to school, developing better relationships and so on.

We actually talk ourselves out of these good ideas, our internal dialogue cheats us, lets us down directing out attention away from the possibilities and into failure or at the very least staying exactly where we are.

I give my clients exercises in rewriting this internal dialogue by having them practice NOT using certain words one of those words is

TRY

We should never try we just do or don't do something

Trying is not succeeding it is attempting and attempting is exactly what it is, an attempt.

How often have you been driving along alone in your thoughts and said I should really try that, I should try to start that business I've always dreamed about

I will try to be better to my husband
I will try to listen to the wife more
I will try to go back to school

Each of these statements sounds positive on the surface yet they are attempts at something, attempts that in most cases never move beyond the initial thought process the actual doing may never happen.

Have you ever thrown party, called friends to invite them and some of those friends use the line ***'Ok I'll try to make it'***

We soon discovered that those are the very people who did not turn up at all.

Have you ever been to a business meeting and said here's a new way we could do this or here's a method we should implement?

Management has replied ***"Oh we tried that and it didn't work"***. When you know full well they didn't.

In couples counselling I often pull many people up when they use the expression such as ***"I'll try that"*** or ***"I'll try to be more open"***.

The word 'try' when attached to any sentence or ***statement of intent*** causes the subconscious mind to believe that you have already done it

If you have done it or attempted it in the past and you failed then why should you do it again, why try again with something that you know (believe) will fail.

I teach my clients to be aware of when they are using the word try both internally and in general conversation, and to listen to others using it, you will be surprised at how often we use it in casual conversation and allow this simple word to redirect our thoughts, feelings and emotions. Once we feel something we are inclined to act on those feelings, and try makes us feel there is little point in pursuing a certain line of action.

There are twelve basic words that have these negative emotional effects on us. I teach clients how to not use them or to realign and reframe that internal dialogue into something more powerful and positive.

The word try however for the moment has another effect that we can use constructively to create change in a person cause them to feel something different and in many cases to act differently.

THE TRY EFFECT

Ask a person to try something and they are unlikely to succeed, this doesn't mean sentences like "try to drink this coffee" will have this effect. Chances are they will drink the coffee and make a fool of your new found mind powers

What it means is a reversal of the natural way we have been trained almost since birth to respond to certain words as in

"Try not to feel better about that"

The old phrase don't think of a hippopotamus is more powerful when delivered with a try

As in

Try not to think of a hippopotamus

Try not to feel happy about this

Try not to agree with me

I've used the following line in weight lose sessions to great effect

Try not to eat more than you can next meal

It's a reverse positive

The brain or mind of the client expects the therapist say something like

Try to eat less next meal

Yet as we have discovered the mind will see this eating less as a failed attempt and may be inclined to eat more, so by reversing it

"Try not to eat more" we are asking them to try and eat less but in reverse.

This effect also comes from the principle that about 90 per cent of the time people 'speak' the opposite of what they 'mean'

You may have had the experience of a person saying 'you can trust me' only to discover later, that this was the first person to break your trust.

Imagine the person who says 'I don't like gossip' then starts an inclement round of telling you all the local news, gossiping, or the person who says 'I'm going to start a business one day' and never does.

Whenever a person says something like this and you believe they are speaking in the opposite, reverse it and create a mind altering sentence that propels them toward their true goals, this is great news for therapists who want to help clients to move forward.

'I'll try to listen to my wife more'

Becomes

'Try to avoid not listening to her'

Powerful stuff, if mixed with the next technique can lead not only to change in others but massive changes in yourself just by realigning your own internal dialogue.

In my stage show I use the concept very effectively, I ask the audience to interlock their fingers leaving the two pointer fingers extended, then have them imagine that the fingertips contain very powerful magnets, which are even now drawing those fingers closer and closer together in fact the harder you try to keep them apart the more powerful that magnetic attraction becomes try harder to keep them apart and notice how they are drawn together until they touch

This psychological illusion relies on a scary fact about human nature, as soon as the mind hears the word "try" it believes that failure is eminent, that the fingers will touch, because they will fail to keep them apart.

As I stated at the beginning of this book, words are incredibly powerful. Even the simplest of phrases has an emotional effect on virtually everyone who hears it; from now on you should be intrinsically aware of this and speak carefully and with intent.

TIME

If you can screw with a person's time line you can alter the way they perceive things, the way they feel about things and the actions they will take concerning those things.

For example we showed how someone who tries to attend your party might not actually attend or are less likely to

So next time this situation occurs do something like this

Don't arrive before seven that's when we open the keg,

Altering time gives a sense of subconscious urgency to a statement and often the need to complete some action.

For example a friend of mine kept leaving messages for a particular business associate and for whatever reason that person failed to return his calls. After a bit of coaching we came up with the following message

'Hi john its Fred just checking in about that contract but please don't call me back before 7 tonight as I'm not available till then
Cheers'
Fred

At 701 pm that night John was on the phone for some reason he felt it necessary even urgent to call back.

We can screw with time in other ways, for example getting the kids to clean their room a mother might say

'Don't clean your rooms before 3 o'clock'

Because they simply want to stir the fat most kids will start cleaning their rooms straight away, naughty aren't they?

Here we are combining the techniques of reverse thinking, time and the try technique all combined into a clever soup that causes people to rethink what they were thinking or even not thinking about a certain thing, then to act on it and act quickly.

Creating sense of urgency is an important and highly effective technique then reverse that sense of urgency makes it doubly powerful.

In therapy I have used such statements to great effect

'Well let's not give up smoking too quickly let's get the body used to it'

Or

'Today is not a good day for you to let go of smoking'
'You don't want to lose weight too fast it can damage your health'.

Don't clean your room too fast take your time

Altering someone's perception of time is an effective way of reconstructing our sentences to have a greater effect on those listening

FILLING IN THE GAPS
THE CHAPTER AFTER THE LAST ONE

Chances are you already knew this was not the last chapter or you may have gone back over the pages and checked what chapter it was, the point is you will have most likely filled in the gap yourself. Most people will fill in caps or attempt to reason out any confusing statements they hear. When this section started you probably got confused and tried to reason it out. During this time other information may have been given to you that you were totally unaware of...

Often people will jump ahead in their reasoning and complete a sentence or statement themselves for example count 1, 2, 3, and your mind is already jumping to 4, 5, and 6

If somebody thinks or feels that something is their own idea or that they made the discovery themselves or joined the dots they are more likely to go along with it.

In therapy the idea was first written about by Carl Rogers as a process of self-discovery or self-healing, where the client would talk and the therapist would listen allowing the client to reach their own conclusions just by asking key questions

Client: '**I don't know what to feel about this**'

Therapist: **Ok what if you did know**

Client: '**Well I'd be sad about it or angry**'

Construct sentences in such a way it allows the listener to fill in the gaps

For example the wife who wants her lawn cut might say

Do we need to use the lawn mower yet?

Another example might be where you ask, Can you imagine situations where you will use these techniques? The listeners mind leaps to situations where they could indeed use these techniques.

What have we learned thus far, we know that we must firstly **know our outcome** don't start talking or using these techniques unless you know what the end result for you is, in fact it is better to know the end result for all parties in a conversation work toward win- win situations,

We have learned that **you really need to shut up**, even if you have the best of intentions in mind somebody is going to get upset if they believe that you are employing any kind of technique to influence them.

Imagine what would happen if somebody stopped you mid conversation and started accusing you of using some sort of hypnotic mind trap, then started blaming you for everything that ever went wrong in their life, it has happened.

And even though religious groups such as fundamentalist movements and even some new age groups use these techniques all the time they frown upon them, deny they use them, and even in some cases say they are the work of the devil.

We have also learned that words have a definite effect on a person's state, it is after all how we communicate, you cannot have an experience in the world and share that experience with me, without using words, the words you chose can help me imagine the experience, feel the terror, share your fun or even taste the food.

THE 'CAN YOU IMAGINE' TECHNIQUE

Asking someone to imagine almost anything actually gets them to imagine that experience or relate the information to something they already know and understand,

Imagine that you've been sky diving and you are trying to relate that experience to a friend who has never jumped out of a perfectly good plane.

At first you might think it's difficult to convey that emotion, that exhilaration yet as you talk and describe the experience your friend seems to understand what you talking about. This is because your friend has been in high places and is extrapolating your story to his own experience and along with you imagining what it would be like.

Asking someone to imagine something is a very powerful technique when done in the right way. During therapy I might ask a couple to imagine what it would be like if a particular problem did not exist or have any influence on their lives.

A classic example is the husband who kept leaving the cap off the tooth paste I asked the wife it was actually important, she said it wasn't it just annoyed her because that's not the way her family had done it.

I then asked if she knew or could imagine anyone who wasn't annoyed by it. She did have a friend who this type of thing didn't seem to bother, I then asked her to imagine what it would be like if she felt the same way about it as her friend,

Moments later that problem didn't exist for her, because by imagining it, she had to bring it into her own awareness, to feel it and wonder what it might be like.

A few of my younger friends spend some time and resources downloading dating manuals from the internet, these manuals by suspiciously named NLP and mind seduction experts, claimed to be able to get the reader more dates more romance even causing women to fall in love with you or become hopelessly attached to the idea of you.

Most of them are a simply reworking of the techniques in this book, the remainder where descriptions of various ways to get your target girl to imagine what it would be like to date you.

So if you are thinking of getting one of these manuals let me save you some time or money

Get someone to imagine the best date, night out or fun time they have ever had then connect that happy memory to you

There you are how easy was that?

Just try not to imagine all the dates you can now get with this technique

Whether it be for dating, self-improvement, motivation or counselling the imagination is one of our most powerful resources, if a person imagines themselves failing at some task the imagination will win every time, so getting them to imagine themselves succeeding is the way to go.

On stage I might use the following phrase *"can you imagine a time when you were so relaxed, so comfortable that you just drifted off into a deep relaxing sleep".*

The phrase is said as part of a larger induction and not really listened to, volunteers are still wondering when I'm going to start hypnotizing them, well guess what I just did.

Often I find myself in situations where people who know what I do, will ask for advice about various problems, perhaps phobias or concerns, at other times they will want to test my supposed hypnotic powers. I meet challenges in a specific way but problems are much easier issue.

First I might ask them to imagine what it would be like if they didn't have that fear, say spiders for example, this is after I check that it is actually a problem and not a simple respect for the fact that they are nasty things that can sneak up on you, but a real life altering fear, like not being able to walk into a room without checking that there are no spiders,

Then I tell them that I'm not going to hypnotize them, probably because we are in the middle of a party or at a restaurant, but I am going to get them to relax for a moment, just deeply enough that I can access the subconscious

I give them a little talk I've developed on this then I hypnotize them even though I have said I'm not going to

One of the first things I will say is

'Just imagine that you are hypnotized, even though you're not actually hypnotised, yet, I want you to imagine or pretend that you are'

To pretend or imagine something, at least a part of you must know what that is like and you will become hypnotized

Be aware I'm not giving away my whole technique here just the imagining part, however the astute reader will notice that the word 'yet" is a specific type of single bind that implies that the subject will become hypnotised, it's just a question of when and how, you are creating an assumption within the subconscious mind.

Ask a child to imagine that they might be a princess or a cowboy and they will have no trouble at all, then ask them to imagine picking up their cloths, job done.

Ask the boss to imagine his business making more sales then ask him to imagine listening to your new ideas, job done.

THE ASKING FOR ADVICE TECHNIQUE

Research shows us that people tend to like you more if they do you a favour not the other way around, we are taught from early childhood that we should be sharing, caring and do favours for people and they will like us.

What we forget is that others have this same programming, they feel that if they are caring and share with us or do us favours that we will like them more, and everybody wants to be liked.

A very good friend of mine had racked up an extraordinary amount of fines. As a young carefree spirit he had avoided paying those fines through a combination of laziness along with being too busy chatting up girls to pay any heed to the impending doom of a fines collector banging on the door, most of us know this bad feeling so he asked me what to do

I suggested he go to the finance company and ask for help. Take the 'what should I do' approach 'you are the experts can you help me', it worked. By dealing with the guy behind the counter as a friend and asking for his help my friend had appealed to that need we all have to be liked

Most people will virtually bend over backwards to do things for you if they believe that you need their help, that it was them that you turned to in your time of need. And all it takes is a simple readjustment of your language,

Yes there are people who relish the power given them in some positions they wrongly feel that they have been given the power of life and death over you, and if you ask them for help they will do everything they can to screw you over, move on ask somebody else for help

Next time you have a problem with large company find out who your contact is and ask for their assistance, tell them that you are lost, don't know what to do, and ask for their advice on what to do. You might even say that they were recommended by someone else, that they are the person to see

Most people will go in at some level of attack or accusation that the company is up to no good or ripping off their customers, the person you speak to on the phone will most likely have been dealing with this attitude all week. If you are polite friendly and actually treating them like they know their job and may actually be able to assist you, not only will they be pleasantly surprised they will go out of their way to help you.

On another occasion I had placed an advertisement in a magazine, at the time I was lead into the ad by a very good and forceful salesman who actively railroaded me into saying yes to the ad,

He actually asked for my help 'because' his magazine did not have a hypnotherapist and they needed one to advertise.

At the time I was stone cold broke and quite honestly unable to pay the extraordinarily large fee, basically I felt that I'd been ripped off

So I reversed the process after many avoided phone calls and not wanting to deal with the matter because I was angry, I decided to at least have a go at what I'd been preaching to my clients, next time they rang demanding money I asked for help

The ad was wrong it did not say I was a hypnotherapist it just said weight loss and my phone number, 'can you help me out what should I do, nobody will call and if they do they will call under the impression that I'm a diet company, I am defiantly going to lose clients through this so I need your help can you work this out for me.

The ad was rewritten and I got the next three instalments for free I did not blame the person ringing and shifted the fault to either the printer or somebody else down the line, I even treated the person on the phone as if they owned the company.

As parents it might be advisable to ask children to help rather than 'clean your room'

Say this

I need your help with some important stuff, and it would help me out if you can clean your room

Treating people like they are experts and asking for their help is an over looked technique that has a power all its own, it builds instant rapport and will solve more issues than you might imagine. Use it

When I first started my radio show, all I had was an idea and a vague hope that I could get it on air, I walked into a radio station which in itself is unusual, and normally they would deal with people through phone or emails.

Standing at the reception desk I said something like the following

'I was just wondering if you could help me you'd be the people to talk to, how do I get a radio show on air, who do I see what should I do'.

Because the show was unusual in its format I would have found it very difficult to describe the concept in written form, to 'sell' it I needed to pitch it, transfer my excitement and passion for the idea in words

The receptionist called a station program manager and he asked what have you got, the rest is history.

Footnote even as I was writing this chapter I applied the technique, by asking people for help, rather than just reading the chapter and telling me what they thought, I said I need you help with this, the result was that even those people who would normally have avoided even the slightest interest in a project that involved reading anything, helped me out by reading the chapter even my laziest of friends rushed to help me by reading the entire manuscript.

BECAUSE

My mother used to ask us some ridiculous things as kids, things like

Clean your room, water the garden, be nice to your sister along with a host of others

Like any kid I would ask why

Just because that's why, was her answer

Had my mother read this book or others like it, she would have known she was only a few words away from an influencing technique that is now famous in psychological circles.

Because technique

Like the previous examples this technique is so powerful when used correctly that what your saying doesn't necessarily have to be true,

I'm not condoning lying what we mean here is that it doesn't have to be relevant to the present situation

The following experiment has been performed in universities all over the world, an office photo copier is organized to be fully booked out people are lined up waiting to use the copier, then another person tries to jump the line, normally this is considered bad form. However when someone says can I jump the line or get ahead of you, because I'm late, or because my mother is on the phone, the whole dynamic is changed, using the word because creates a plausible reason within the mind of the listener.

"just sit in the chair because it will help you to relax' is not true, a certain chair will not make you relax any more effectively than any other chair, yet the sentence seems to make sense.

A PERSON MIGHT

We spoke before about tags and how the most important tag you can use is the person's name. It creates focus and virtually forces the attention of the mind to what comes next, since early childhood we have been indirectly programmed to respond to our names.

A sentence or statement can still have power if your name is not directly at the beginning depending on the way a statement is formed, and of course depending on what you want your message to be.

The a person might tag can be placed in front of a name to give it more internal power, giving the statement a slight authority shift,

'A person might John, take the lessons of today and be able to let go of the past'

In therapy this is a powerful technique especially when attached to a deep meaningful metaphor about healing the pains we still carry with us from past experiences,

'A person might Mary be able to let go of the anger and listen to another's point of view'

We could even shorten this

'A person might Mary be able to see this from another point of view'

Like some of our other tags this also provides you with an out in some situations, you are not saying that Mary can do this you are simply stating that someone might be able to.

In most cases however this tag in a statement will cause an authority shift 'if someone else can then perhaps I can to'.

In therapy I will use a CHC in the second part of the statement in the example of weight lose I might say something to the effect of

'A person might Sarah find a reason to make losing weight actually seem like fun'

When delivered correctly in a casual almost throw away manner this is a very powerful statement, the hidden command was

'You will find a reason to make losing weight fun'

It was hidden in the rest of the statement and is able to slip in past the conscious reasoning, or that part of the mind that rejects the idea of losing weight as being fun, in fact in most cases we naturally believe that losing weight is not fun at all.

However we now have a sense that or believe that some other person has found it fun and there is no reason to think that you couldn't as well.

This is a powerful tag and like others you should practice it once the opportunity arises or a situation occurs where you feel that it is suitable.

CAN YOU IMAGINE SITUATIONS WHERE YOU WILL USE THESE TECHNIQUES?

What have we learned thus far, we know that we must firstly know our outcome don't start talking or using these techniques unless you know what the end result for you is, in fact it is better to know the end result for all parties in a conversation work toward win- win situations,

We have learned that you really need to shut up, even if you have the best of intentions in mind somebody is going to get upset if they believe that you are employing any kind of technique to influence them.

Imagine what would happen if somebody stopped you mid conversation and started accusing you of using some sort of hypnotic mind trap, then started blaming you for everything that ever went wrong in their life, it has happened.

And even though religious groups such as fundamentalist Christian movements and even some new age groups use these techniques all the time they frown upon them, deny they use them, and even in some cases say they are the work of the devil.

We have also learned that words have a definite effect on a person's state, it is after all how we communicate, you cannot have an experience in the world and share that experience with me, without using words, the words you chose can help me imagine the experience, feel the terror, share your fun or even taste the food.

Well I Hope You Enjoyed This Small Journey Into The World Of Erotic And Covert Hypnosis. As much as I enjoyed writing it My Final Advice...Practise and Enjoy...